ECZE

AND OTHER SKIN DISORDERS

ECZEMA

AND OTHER SKIN DISORDERS

The self-care guide

DR JOVANKA BACH

GRAFTON BOOKS

A Division of the Collins Publishing Group

LONDON GLASGOW
TORONTO SYDNEY AUCKLAND

Grafton Books
A division of the Collins Publishing Group
8 Grafton Street, London W1X 3LA

Published by Grafton Books 1987

British Library Cataloguing in Publication Data

Bach, Jovanka
    Eczema and other skin disorders: the self-care guide.
    1. Skin – Diseases – Treatment
    2. Self-care, Health
    I. Title
    616.5'068   RL111

    ISBN 0-246-12947-6

Photoset in Linotron Electra by
Rowland Phototypesetting Ltd,
Bury St Edmunds, Suffolk
Printed in Great Britain by
Robert Hartnoll (1985), Bodmin

CONTENTS

INTRODUCTION: WHAT IS ECZEMA?

Many things in Western civilization stem from the Greeks, and eczema is no exception. The Greeks coined the word; it means 'boil out'. Eczema first begins as small blisters, resembling sago or tapioca granules. Thus, to the Greeks, the skin appeared to be 'bubbling' or 'boiling out'.

The condition is certainly an old one – probably as old as man. It is also quite common. Up to half of the British population will have it at one time or another, and 25 per cent of patients attending hospital skin clinics come in for treatment of eczema.

Eczema itches – almost always. If it does not itch, we can assume the condition is not eczema. In most people's minds it is associated with a specific and major skin disease – atopic eczema, which can affect a person at any point in his or her life from infancy (infantile eczema) to adulthood. It is hereditary and often associated with hay fever, asthma and/or hives.

But eczema is not just atopic eczema. The term is used, in a broader context, to refer to a range of eczema-type patterns, or 'reaction-patterns', common to several skin diseases, each of which has a different and in many cases unknown origin. (I shall discuss these, as well as atopic eczema, in the following chapters.) This dual meaning has created ambiguity and confusion in communication between doctors, and between doctor and patient.

Semantics have always plagued dermatologists, never more so than in eczema. To clear up the confusion surrounding this term, the word 'dermatitis' was introduced, meaning 'inflammation of the dermis' (the second or supporting layer of the skin). Many dermatologists prefer this term, saying it describes the abnormal process of inflammation (dilated skin vessels with surrounding influx of white cells) that occurs in eczema conditions. However, purists point out that skin eruptions of many kinds show inflammation in the dermis. Therefore, 'dermatitis' is really a nonspecific and general term. Nevertheless, the term began to be used as a substitute and interchangeable word for eczema. Therefore, it is now used not only to describe eczema, but also in a more general sense to identify other skin conditions. For example, drug eruptions are also called, medically, *dermatitis medicamentosa.*

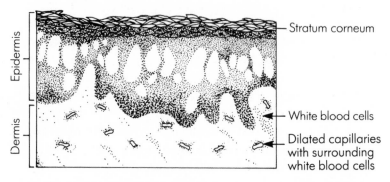

Fig.1 *Acute dermatitis as seen under the microscope,* when a piece of tissue (biopsy) is taken for processing and examination. Many changes are taking place in the skin, primarily in the top layer, known as the epidermis. The latter is also divided into layers. Its top layer, the stratum corneum, is more scaly than usual. The spaces in the middle layer, the stratum spinosum, correspond to the blisters that we see on the skin. These blisters contain tissue fluid and sometimes white cells.

In the second skin layer, the dermis, dilated capillaries, with their accompanying white blood cells and tissue fluid (oedema), cause the redness and swelling that we see in the skin with the naked eye.

Purists and ambiguity aside, some order has to prevail. In this book, I shall follow the accepted practice of most skin doctors, using 'dermatitis' in preference to 'eczema'. When I do use the word 'eczema', as it is hard to get away from it, I use it basically in the specific sense, to mean atopic eczema. If I use the word otherwise, I shall qualify it so you will know what I am writing about.

Since the operative word is dermatitis, the three stages by which it manifests itself will be known as acute, subacute and chronic dermatitis. These are the typical prototype reactions that identify this dermatitis group, and should be remembered.

Tiny, itchy blisters on a red, slightly to moderately swollen skin surface characterize the early *acute* stage (Fig. 1). If treatment is not begun immediately, this soon progresses to the *subacute* stage. The skin over the blisters becomes scaly and breaks, and oozing and crusted red patches develop. Infection can occur because the crusts and body fluid are good breeding substances for bacteria. The *chronic* stage develops when eczema is not treated promptly or adequately, or when the condition continues over a period of time with repeated clearing and recurrence.

The distinguishing features in chronic eczema are dry, scaly thickening with prominent skin markings (lichenification) (Figs. 2 and 3). The latter gives an 'elephant-hide' look to the involved area, which is now called a 'plaque' because of its thicker, drier, more defined appearance. Redness of the underlying and surrounding skin may or may not be part of the picture.

A darkening of the plaque may occur. This is due to disruption of the pigment-forming cells (melanocytes) that exist in the bottom layer of the epidermis (Fig. 5). Repeated inflammation provokes them to release pigment into the lower layer of the skin, the dermis. This pigment (melanin) gives the plaque a tan or slightly dusky colour.

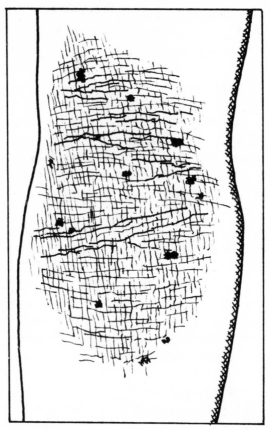

Fig. 2 Chronic dermatitis with scratch marks. This is in an elbow crease, as typically seen in atopic dermatitis. The 'elephant hide' appearance of the skin, with accentuated skin markings, is apparent. There is also dryness and more scaling than in acute dermatitis.

The three stages are by no means distinctly separated from each other. It is not unusual to see one stage evolving into another, or for all three stages to be present, especially in a chronic eczema which has flared up. Scratch and gouge marks are common too. They are a reaction to the severe itching which usually accompanies eczema.

Despite its prevalence, many aspects of dermatitis are

misunderstood or not understood at all. It is difficult to study because it is a reaction-pattern to an underlying process and too many factors are in play at one time. Research thrives best where there is an orderly, well-defined process. Thus, in the dermatitis group, sophisticated research tools have yet to give us adequate answers.

Since more than one disease may precipitate the dermatitis reaction, doctors may have trouble deciding which one is causal. Therefore, they are likely to lump the diagnosis under the term 'eczema' or 'dermatitis', and be vague in their explanation to you, the patient. You may go away discontented, with diminished confidence in your physician. Questions will whirl in your head: 'How can the doctor help me if he doesn't know what I have?', 'And what about the medicine he prescribed? Will it do me any good?'

Perhaps you will slack off on the medicine, not sure that it will help anyway. And since you are not applying the preparations as needed, they will not do much good. You will

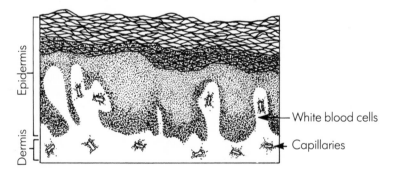

Fig. 3 Chronic dermatitis as seen under the microscope. The epidermis shows a thickened top layer, and few, if any, blisters in its middle layer. This corresponds to the thick, scaly, dry appearance of the dermatitis as viewed by the naked eye. The dilated capillaries and white cells in the dermis contribute to the reddish and swollen look of the dermatitis clinically.

feel frustrated, and may develop the hopeless attitude of 'Why bother?'

But you *should* bother. Your general well-being depends on it, and dermatitis is really not so complicated. In the following chapters, I hope to make sense of it; to break it down into the various types, describing and defining them so that you have a better understanding of what it is that you have, and how best to treat it.

Based on causative factors, the dermatitis group has been divided into two major categories: internal and external. This provides a point of reference and facilitates better understanding of the various dermatitis conditions.

This book is devoted to a discussion of diseases under these two headings, with information and advice about other relevant skin conditions. I hope you will find it informative and helpful, and that it clarifies some of the misconceptions and confusion about eczema – or dermatitis.

Chapter One

THE SKIN: ITS FUNCTIONS

What is the largest organ in the body? It is the skin. That information may come as a surprise, especially if you haven't bothered to think about it. Or, maybe, even if you have.

The skin is a vital organ – certainly we could not survive without it. Severe second- and third-degree burns can bring us to death's door. And extensive sunburn can change the temperature control in the skin and make us chilled and sick, as can rashes that mimic sunburn.

The skin is not just a surface organ. It is closely related, physiologically and biochemically, with the rest of your body. Your skin is a mirror of your health. If you are exhausted, have a cold or are anaemic, your skin will show it. Are you a heavy, long-term smoker? Most likely your face will have many fine, puckered wrinkles. Or do you drink heavily? Your face will show small blood vessels on the nose, cheeks and upper chest – or you may develop a W. C. Fields nose, but not necessarily his humour.

As a dermatologist, it is interesting for me to travel on the underground and observe people – discreetly, of course, from behind a newspaper. On their faces are spots, dilated vessels, cracks at the corners of their mouths and other signs of their states of health and habits. Fortunately, most people that I observe are perfectly healthy, and their good skin texture and tone reflect this.

Anatomy of the Skin

Two layers comprise the skin – the top layer, the epidermis, and the thicker layer beneath it, the dermis (Fig. 4). The epidermis is our outer coat, our protection and barrier against injury. Its cells manufacture keratin which functions in this protection. Irritation or damage to the epidermis will make us more vulnerable to noxious topical chemicals. (A word about keratin: it is a complex protein substance that makes up skin scales. A specialized form of keratin forms hair and nails.)

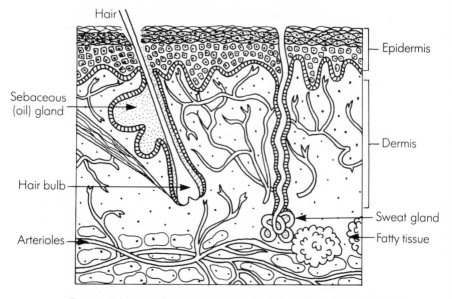

Fig. 4 Schematic Representation of the Skin as Seen Microscopically.
The top layer is the epidermis. In itself it consists of several layers (see Fig. 5).

The second layer, the dermis, provides support and gives the skin its stretch and flexibility. The dermis contains the smooth muscle of the hair, the oily (sebaceous) gland, as well as a complex of fine nerves and vessels. The hair structure, known as the hair follicle, and the sweat gland originate in the dermis, near the underlying fatty tissue. This subcutaneous layer cushions the skin. Larger vessels, which course through it, supply the skin with nutrients.

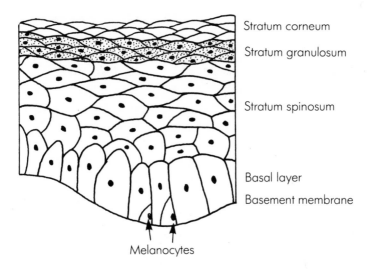

Stratum corneum

Stratum granulosum

Stratum spinosum

Basal layer

Basement membrane

Melanocytes

Fig. 5   Microscopic Diagram of the Epidermis (Upper Skin Layer). As seen in Fig. 4, four layers comprise the epidermis, which is separated from the dermis by a submicroscopic basement membrane. The basal cells give rise to the other epidermal cells, which progressively evolve to form the scaly, top stratum corneum. The granules in the stratum granulosum, the second layer, function actively in scale formation.

The melanocytes do not originate from basal cells, but migrate to the epidermis during foetal formation.

The *epidermis* itself is divided into several layers (see Fig. 5). The junction between epidermis and dermis is marked by a membrane of fine submicroscopic fibres, called the basement membrane. Above it is the bottom basal layer of the epidermis, which contains the germ cells (basal cells) that produce the rest of the epidermis. Their course is progressively towards more and more keratin formation through the second middle layer, the stratum spinosum, which consists of several cells, through a thinner granular layer, and finally to the scaly acellular top layer, the stratum corneum. This is the scaly skin surface that sheds, with new cells continually replacing it.

15

Melanocytes, the pigment-forming cells in the epidermis, determine our ability to tan and our skin colour. They occupy sites between the basal cells of the bottom layer. When they are damaged, as in dermatitis, they release pigment into the underlying dermis. The skin then shows increased pigmentation, which is reversible as the problem improves.

The *dermis* is richly supplied with blood vessels and nerve fibres. The former carry nutrients to the skin and function in temperature control. The latter supply sensation. Sweat glands, oil (sebaceous) glands and hair also arise in the dermis and find their way to the skin's surface by ducts. Collagen and elastic fibres in the dermis provide the skin with its elasticity and pliability.

The skin is not the same everywhere on the body. It varies in thickness and texture, depending on localized function. On the lips and genital areas it is modified and called semi-mucous membrane. The cells contain some mucus and form little keratin, with the resultant absence of the outer scaly layer. The skin here is shiny, smoother and softer to the touch than skin on other body parts. It is also more sensitive.

The thickness of the skin depends in some areas on the epidermis and in others on the dermis. On the palms and soles, the epidermis is very thick and protects from irritation and penetration of chemicals. On the back and scalp, the dermis is quite thick – providing protection from physical injury.

Oil, sweat glands and hair vary in degree in different parts of the body. Although found everywhere, sweat glands are particularly abundant on the palms, the soles, in the armpits, and on the back, scalp and forehead.

Oil glands are usually found in association with hair, and are most common in the areas of the head and face. They do not occur on the palms and soles. Specialized oil glands exist in the ear canal and genital area, and specialized sweat glands, the apocrine, are likewise found in the genital region and in the armpits.

The location of regular hair is obvious, but fine (lanugo) hair exists all over our bodies, and aids in touch and sensation.

Basic Physiology

The skin protects us. It shields our inner organs from chemical and physical damage. It keeps many harmful chemicals from entering our bodies, but bear in mind that any noxious substance should always be washed off immediately, since exposure for any length of time increases the risk of penetration and/or skin damage.

In addition to keeping noxious substances out, the skin also keeps salt and water inside the body. This barrier against external chemicals and internal biochemicals can change and break down when there is extensive inflammation or blistering of the skin, as is present in dermatitis and burns. Then liquids can leak out and be lost, creating problems with the body's fluid balance. Damaged skin no longer has its protective shield. External substances can penetrate and contact allergies are more likely to develop.

The barrier also breaks down when the skin is made soggy from immersion in water for too long, or when rubber gloves or shoes are worn which create sweat and subsequent maceration of the surface layer. This skin alteration is used to advantage in the treatment of chronic dermatitis. Here, cortisone medication applied under plastic occlusion, which promotes moisture, penetrates faster than when applied to a dry surface.

The skin contains many elastic and collagen fibres. These make it pliable and plastic, permitting quite a bit of stretching or pulling. This elasticity of the skin gives physical protection from shearing and stretching types of pressure. Since collagen and elastic fibres decrease with age, the protective resilience of the skin also diminishes.

We feel and touch with our skin, as well as experience pain, heat and cold. An abundance of sensory organs in the skin absorb these sensations. We experience them in the brain after they have been conducted to it through a complicated system of interconnected nerve fibres.

A crucial function of the skin is temperature control. This is maintained by an abundant supply of small blood vessels and capillaries, and by sweat glands. Under nervous system control, blood vessels become wider (dilate) to accommodate an increased blood flow to the skin, and conversely, become more narrow (constrict) to decrease blood flow. This dilatation and expansion of vessels controls blood flow and, therefore, heat loss or heat conservation. Since blood is a medium for conducting body heat, increased blood flow increases heat loss through the skin, and decreased flow decreases heat loss.

In hot weather, the sweat (eccrine) glands start working when the blood flow method cannot adequately cool down the body, and in very hot weather, sweat evaporation becomes the most important mechanism for temperature control.

Normal physiological functions are necessary to preserve the integrity of the skin. When they falter, skin diseases appear. For example, in atopic dermatitis, sweating and temperature-regulating mechanisms are not normal. The blood vessels do not respond in the usual way to heat and cold. Certain parts of the body, i.e. toes, fingers and nose, are colder than in people who do not have this condition. Although the significance of this difference is not yet apparent, decreased sweating in atopic dermatitis is known to contribute to dryness and severe itching.

The pigment-forming cells, melanocytes, located in the bottom layer of the epidermis, protect us from the damaging rays of the sun. These cells form a pigment, melanin, which is dispersed throughout the epidermis and absorbs harmful rays. A short exposure to the sun will trigger these cells to form more pigment. A tan develops slowly over a period of time, and the increased pigment or melanin gives us protection from the damaging burning rays.

The fat film which exists on the skin's surface plus the resident community of non-infectious bacteria and fungi help to protect us from infections. These organisms somehow work together to suppress the growth of dangerous infective organisms. The thin surface fat (or lipid) layer further aids this process, and also acts as a barrer to certain chemicals and water. When this lipid layer is stripped away, by solvents for example, the skin becomes more susceptible to irritation. This increases the risk of contact dermatitis which can be a problem in certain industries (see Chapter 3).

Chapter Two

INTERNAL GROUP
or 'Blame it on
Grandpa'

ATOPIC DERMATITIS

Atopic dermatitis is a familial or genetically-influenced itchy skin rash, with which asthma, hay fever and hives are associated, either in the patient or in members of the patient's family. Most patients have only the dermatitis, but about 30 per cent may have one or more of the other associated conditions. If not, there is usually a family history of someone – a brother, sister, aunt, uncle – with asthma, hay fever or hives.

If you have atopic dermatitis, you may have developed it first during infancy. Here it starts at about the age of two months, and by the age of two years is often gone. At times it may persist through childhood, but in a modified form (see below). Unlike adult dermatitis, it may be associated with food allergies to cow's milk, cheese, eggs and wheat. These foods make the rash worse and have to be avoided. Fortunately, food allergies as a causative factor of the dermatitis disappear as the child grows up. In adult atopics ingested foods play little, if any, role in dermatitis, although certain foods have been implicated in the production of hives. Infantile eczema will not be a focus of discussion here, as it has been well covered in other books.

Alternatively, you may have developed the eczema during childhood and have skipped the infant phase. Here the rash is drier. It may still go through an acute phase with tiny blisters or vesicles, but it does not persist as long in this stage. The presentation is more likely to be as drier, firmer vesicles which combine to form scaly, itchy red patches, primarily on the flexor surfaces of the body (see Fig. 6). The flexor surfaces are those in the bends of the elbows, fronts of the forearms, behind the knees and on the calves. This distribution is typical for atopic dermatitis in all its stages and helps to distinguish it from other eczemas. However, in infantile eczema, face and nappy involvement are often predominant over flexor involvement.

You may survive the childhood phase to be left with the sole problem of dry skin. Or the rash may come and go into adulthood.

Sometimes atopic dermatitis does not appear until adolescence or adulthood. You may, however, have noticed that your skin was always drier than normal, or that you were plagued with hay fever symptoms at certain times of the year. Possibly, you may have developed hives when you got upset or over-exerted yourself. Asthma may have been a problem. And someone in your family may have had the atopic tendencies. Or maybe not.

Indicators of atopy, as the overall genetic state is called, are not always evident. You may have had no more than some dryness of your skin to which you paid no attention. Then one day you erupt into an excruciatingly itchy rash. There are other markers. However, you would not know about them unless you were very knowledgeable about atopic dermatitis. For one, a specific horizontal crease may be present on the palms. And there is an extra fold under the lower eyelids. This 'Mongolian' fold, as it is called, is peculiar to patients with the atopic rash.

Other findings include coldness of the distal parts of the body, particularly the toes, fingers and end of the nose. You will be sensitive to temperature changes, especially sudden,

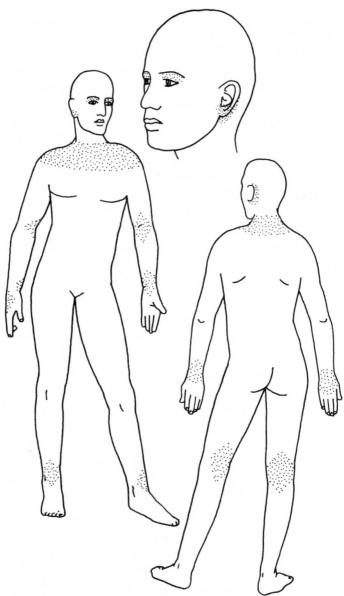

Fig. 6 Atopic Dermatitis — Characteristic Locations. These are primarily in creases (flexural), although the back of the neck, upper chest, eyelids and earlobes are common locations. Compare to Psoriasis, Fig. 9.

extreme ones. And you will notice you have trouble sweating. Your skin will be drier under emotional pressure and in heat than normal skin.

You may have a greater number of colds than your non-rashy friends. The incidence of pneumonia is 10 to 15 per cent greater than in people without atopic dermatitis. This statistic probably reflects the situation of those patients who have asthma co-existing with their rash.

Doctors have also observed that adult patients have a diminished ability to develop contact allergies, in contrast to individuals with normal skin.

The clinical findings of cooler digits, sensitivity to temperature changes, difficulty in sweating, decreased sensitivity to contact allergies and increased susceptibility to infection led medical investigators to look for internal reasons for these findings.

Biochemical tests showed, in fact, that internal abnormalities are present. An immunoglobulin, IgE, a protein present in certain immune conditions, is elevated in 15 to 30 per cent of patients with atopic dermatitis, but is present in only one per cent of normal patients. When skin is tested with DNCB (dinitrochlorobenzene), a highly potent skin sensitizer, there is a weak reaction, if any, in atopic dermatitis. This chemical causes allergic skin rash in nearly all normal patients. But atopic patients have some defect, as yet undiscovered, in their immune biochemistry, which prevents the usual skin eruption to DNCB.

Other tests showed an abnormality in blood vessel (vascular) response in the skin to heat and cold, and an abnormality in the sweating system.

Based on their findings, medical researchers have proposed two theories of origin for atopic dermatitis. One group supports an immunological theory because of the discoveries of altered immune response. Another group supports a defect in the special nervous system interaction with sweat glands and skin blood vessels. Neither of these theories has enough facts to back it up, and both are quite speculative.

What does this uncertainty about the cause of atopic dermatitis mean for you, the patient? Basically, it means that there is no specific cure or prevention, since the exact cause is not known. At best we can control it, and you have to learn to live with the fact that atopic dermatitis can be a chronic disease that comes and goes.

However, it is not a disease that causes disfigurement or death. It gradually lessens in onset and severity as you approach your thirties and forties, and is not a great problem in the older years. It does not have to be chronic. You may have only one flare-up and no more, or just a brief time period when you are troubled with it.

Much can be done to ease the discomfort from the rash and to decrease the flare-ups. Hydrocortisone and its more potent cousins, the fluorinated steroids, have revolutionized the treatment of atopic dermatitis and made most other topicals obsolete. These medications relieve itching very quickly and soon clear the eruption. They are discussed fully in the section on treatment.

Triggers

Stress is probably the most important factor in triggering an eruption in adult eczema. When you have a row with your girlfriend or boyfriend, or feel pressured by the boss, you will usually break out. Even good stresses, such as getting married, transferring to a better job or to a new house can trigger a rash.

You, the atopic dermatitis patient, are often described as tense, highly ambitious and driven to the point of exhaustion. Some doctors say you may have much repressed hostility, which 'bubbles out' on your skin rather than through constructive means of expression. To this I say: 'Leave off!' There are many tense, driven people who do not have atopic dermatitis. The itching, aggravation and frustration you experience from the dermatitis is enough to make anyone tense, nervous – even hostile. To what degree the psychological and physical affect each other cannot be ascertained. Furthermore, stress can trigger the eruption of many skin diseases other than atopic dermatitis. It also can produce other physical ailments such as migraine, ulcer and high blood pressure, to name a few.

The basic thing to remember is that stress is especially harmful to people who are prone to the development of physical ailments. If you are in a muddle about your life, ask the general practitioner or skin doctor to refer you to a counsellor or counselling clinic. If work or family life is getting you down, take a weekend off. Even a Sunday outing is good relief from daily worry. Learn methods of relaxation: take fifteen minutes twice a day to sit in a quiet room and let your mind wander to some beautiful moment or place that makes you feel good when you think about it (see Chapter 9).

Excessive bathing, especially in hot water, and the use of alkali soaps can irritate your sensitive skin and provoke a reaction; as can woollen fabrics or polyester synthetics that have been treated with formaldehyde to make them wrinkle-resistant. Household cleaners can irritate your skin, as can solvents used in dissolving grease. If you work on your car, be careful not to use solvents to clean your hands; instead, use an emulsifying ointment such as aqueous cream (see List 1, pages 45–8). If you are in contact with solvents or irritating chemicals in your job, your rash may be triggered or aggravated. This may even become an occupational problem if contact is not effectively eliminated (see Chapter 3).

Temperatures that are either too cold or too hot will aggravate your dermatitis. In cold weather, the skin tends to become drier and more chapped. This will cause irritation and itching of the skin with subsequent breaking out.

Because you do not sweat properly, this normal method

for cooling off in hot weather does not work for you. Therefore, heat can be not only uncomfortable, but almost unbearable. Heat plus diminished sweating will produce almost intolerable itching, with subsequent skin eruption. To stop the itching, some people not only scratch but resort to pinching and slapping themselves – often causing black and blue marks – preferring the pain to itching. Obviously you must avoid heat. Wear loose, comfortable clothing. Take cool or at the most tepid showers or baths. Bathing should be quick – just enough to wash off. Prolonged exposure to water, if not followed by application of creams or oils, can dry the skin further.

Interestingly, the beach is helpful to atopic dermatitis. The relaxation of being away, the cooling effect of sea breezes, the healing effect of the sun and the salt water all combine in a beneficial way to clear the eczema. Paradoxically, salt water, which might be expected to be an irritant, turns out to be helpful when the contact is through ocean bathing.

Food allergies (those from eating certain foods) seldom exacerbate adult eczema, although, as mentioned, they do provoke infantile eczema. However, if you cook and get juices from foods such as tomatoes, lemons, oranges and cucumbers on your hands, your skin undoubtedly will get irritated and break out.

Infections

As mentioned earlier, patients with atopic dermatitis are at higher risk of developing infections such as colds and pneumonias. But there is also an increase in skin infections as compared with people with normal skin. The bacterial infections, usually caused by *Staphylococcus aureus*, a common infective organism, primarily affect the oozing, crusting acute and subacute stage, or begin in the scratches and gouges of any stage. Body fluids and crusts are good culture media for bacteria.

Patients with atopic dermatitis are especially susceptible to the viral infections of Herpes Simplex Type I and Vaccinia. Herpes Simplex I causes cold or fever sores, most commonly in body parts above the waist. Vaccinia is the virus of smallpox vaccination. Once established, these can quickly spread to cause a generalized vesicular, viral skin eruption, whether the patient has an active rash at the time or is in a state of remission. The individual may be quite sick, with systemic symptoms of fever, headache and malaise.

Patients should not be vaccinated and should avoid people who have been recently vaccinated and those who have herpes infections. Practically, contact with the vaccinia virus should not be a concern, since the World Health Organization has announced the world-wide eradication of smallpox and no longer considers the vaccination necessary except in unusual circumstances. However, you should guard against herpes infections, which are more prevalent than they were in the past.

Associated finding: 8 per cent of patients with atopic dermatitis will develop cataracts, usually in one eye. Women in their thirties are most susceptible to this. The reasons for this development are unknown.

Complications

Three major complications can occur in atopic dermatitis. They are infection, autosensitization reaction and erythroderma (also known as generalized exfoliative dermatitis). These last two sound like bizarre and incomprehensible processes, but they are not. I will explain them to you shortly.

Infection. Some degree of superficial infection is present

27

in many eczemas, especially the acute and subacute stages and where there are scratch marks and gouges. The skin barrier is violated by oozing blisters and scratches. The body liquids that are brought to the surface are rich in proteins and other nutrients, thus providing an excellent incubator for surface bacteria. When the moist, acute phase is treated quickly with appropriate cleansing agents and topical medications, the superficial infection will clear or be aborted. Internal antibiotics may not even be needed.

The problem arises when the moist dermatitis is inadequately treated, and surface bacteria are allowed to thrive in the oozing rash. The infection will be seen as pus in the blisters or scratch areas, and will spread to the surrounding skin. A red, hot, uncomfortable area with diffuse borders will occur around the patch of dermatitis, or a red streak will begin to go upwards away from it. Either of these changes should propel you at once to your doctor or the nearest emergency clinic for treatment. The appearance of a red streak is especially worrisome. It means the infection is in the lymphatic system and is being carried into the body. It is a good warning signal; it could lead to 'blood poisoning' or blood-borne bacterial infection, and means you will need immediate internal antibiotics.

Lymph nodes draining the involved area will swell. You will feel them as rubbery, almond-shaped knots. If the dermatitis is on the arm, you may feel them around the elbow or in the armpit. If the dermatitis is on the face or head, you will feel them under the jaw, chin or in the back of the neck.

By themselves, swollen lymph glands in dermatitis do not mean you have an infection. If you have had a rash for a while, the glands will swell as a reaction to the biochemical processes going on in the dermatitis. These glands are usually minimally tender, if at all. However, if a tender swollen gland suddenly appears, have it checked by a doctor. It may mean the start of an early infection, and should be appropriately treated. A tender swollen gland may appear before significant pus, spreading redness or a red streak. Noticing it and getting treatment will help abort a more progressive infection.

As a word of caution, I would like to point out that any lump or swelling which you find, regardless of what you think it is, should be checked by a doctor.

Fever and chills are, of course, the signs of an advanced infection which has spread from your skin into your blood stream. This is seen most often in patients with an extensive excoriated (scratched) dermatitis that has not been treated properly. In any case, get medical help immediately.

Autosensitization reaction. In dermatology, this term means a skin rash which results from a sensitivity, literally to oneself. In fact, it is not a sensitivity to oneself but rather to one's chronic skin rash. Patients with any type of dermatitis, not just atopic dermatitis, can develop this reaction which is a rash occurring near the site of the original dermatitis or elsewhere on the body – usually the trunk. The rash often does not have the same appearance as the eczema which initiated it. This is the way the process works.

The autosensitivity rashes do not occur in acute dermatitis, but rather in a more chronic phase which has subsequently become irritated, or in which one portion is flaring up into an acute or subacute phase. The complicated mechanism of skin allergy is at work here, in this case from an internal source rather than from an exterior contactant in the environment.

In acute dermatitis, various substances – proteins, enzymes, prostaglandins – are released into the body from the breakdown of skin cells. The proteins of these breakdown products stimulate the body's immune system to form antibodies. Since the proteins come from skin cells, the antibodies are therefore antagonistic to the skin. Not everyone's immune system reacts in the same way; there are many variables. Some people do not form auto- (self-) antibodies easily; others readily form them.

The skin antibodies, which are special proteins, do not cause trouble if the acute phase is treated and clears. The potential for an autosensitivity rash exists when the initial dermatitis goes into a subacute or chronic phase.

In the untreated subacute phase, skin cells continue to break down and release proteins which stimulate the further formation of antibodies, until a point is reached where these antibodies cause a secondary reaction or rash in the skin.

In chronic dermatitis, there is relatively minimal cellular destruction with release of substances into the body. Therefore the body's immune system remains torpid. When the chronic rash flares into an acute or subacute phase, either from stress, topical irritants or secondary infection, protein by-products of deteriorating skin cells are again dumped into the circulation.

The immune system, which has already been primed by an earlier acute or subacute dermatitis, now makes more antagonistic antibodies, until a level is reached at which the antibodies react with uninvolved skin to form a secondary rash. This is called an autosensitivity reaction.

Medical knowledge about autosensitivity is incomplete. Once geneticists, immunologists and biochemists unravel this complex process, they will unlock secrets of immunology and of dermatitis itself.

The autosensitivity rash usually first occurs contiguous to the original rash. The trunk and hands are most commonly affected when the rash erupts at a site away from the initial dermatitis. Then the patient is often perplexed by the appearance of a new rash which seems unrelated to the original one; more so, since the secondary rash does not resemble the original. Usually it appears as a measles-like rash or as tiny red bumps (papules or vesicles, from 1 to 4 mm in size). These may start as discrete lesions, but soon coalesce to form red, scaly patches. When those occur near the original dermatitis, they may merge with it to form a large local area of involvement. On the palms, soles and sides of the fingers and toes, the autosensitivity reaction may appear as blisters.

The autosensitivity rash means that the eczema is out of control. An internal immune process is at work, which must be stymied if the dermatitis is to resolve. Topical therapy is ineffective. Autosensitivity is one of the indications for the use of systemic cortisones or steroids in atopic dermatitis.

If the autosensitivity rash is not controlled it will progress, as will the eczema – the two merging to produce a much more serious complication – erythroderma.

Erythroderma. This word literally means 'red skin'. A term skin doctors like is 'generalized exfoliative dermatitis', which means a general inflammation of the skin with shredding (exfoliation).

You may have noticed that dermatologists as a group use difficult-sounding Latin names for skin diseases. This is a historical carry-over. When doctors became aware of skin diseases as a fit subject for study, Latin was the pre-eminent scientific language. Since the skin is easily accessible, the early skin doctors were able to examine and name many skin diseases and their variants. Descriptive, diagnostic names were coined, based almost entirely on the appearance of the skin. Unfortunately, many have no relevance to the actual cause of the disease. Dermatology is still hamstrung by this outdated terminology, although attempts are being made to rename diseases according to modern concepts. Enough progress has not been made in this direction, so I shall explain the Latin terms as we go along.

Generalized exfoliative dermatitis, although a mouthful, describes more accurately than 'erythroderma' the total body involvement that can complicate atopic dermatitis. This serious stage of the disease occurs when something aggravates a pre-existing dermatitis, i.e. irritants or localized infection.

It is seen more often in patients of middle age or older. This condition is not confined to dermatitis, but may occur as a complication of other skin diseases such as psoriasis. Rarely, it may develop without an antecedent skin disease, be unresponsive to therapy and become chronic. In these instances it might be a presenting sign of an underlying lymphoma or leukemia. Then, a proper medical work-up is in order to rule out this infrequent but serious possibility.

The skin becomes red and and shiny in appearance. There is a rapid turnover of skin cell formation with constant shedding or flaking away of the stratum corneum, whose absence produces the shiny appearance. The patient's clothes and bed are full of white skin scales. Much blood is shunted through the innumerable dilated blood vessels in the skin, accounting for the redness and creating an increased vascular skin flow. In elderly patients with weak hearts, this increased circulation through the skin can actually produce what is known as high output heart failure. This is aided by a drop in the body protein because of excessive shedding of epidermal scales. They are rich in protein, which the body often cannot manufacture fast enough to keep up with the loss. The result is blood of lower density which circulates faster and further stresses compromised hearts.

With the loss of the surface epidermal layer, the skin's protective mechanisms are literally shed away. The temperature control system suffers: an immense amount of heat is lost through the skin because of the increased blood flow and loss of a protective layer. The patient gets chilled easily, even when it is warm.

Another problem is the easy penetration of bacteria through the denuded skin surface. Thus, these patients are at high risk of internal infections.

Extensive involvement may affect the face and head with loss of eyelashes, eyebrows, even scalp hair. Fortunately this is reversible once the disease is brought under control.

Because of the changes within it (oedema, inflammation and absent protective stratum corneum), the skin becomes taut, especially on the face. This often causes a pulling down of the lower eyelid (called ectropion), which exposes the eye to irritation and produces a compensatory tearing.

Generalized exfoliative dermatitis is fortunately an infrequent complication of atopic dermatitis. If it does happen, hospitalization is indicated, with bed rest, an adequate high-protein diet, soothing baths and emollients to the skin. Internal antibiotics will be needed to counteract infection. Appropriate eye-drops will help relieve eye irritation. Since the dermatitis is very itchy, antihistamines, tranquillizers and even sedatives may need to be taken internally.

The drug of choice for treatment is a steroid by mouth. Prednisone, 40 to 60 mg per day, will usually produce a rapid remission. Once this happens, the patient has to be tapered off the drug gradually, in order to prevent flares which can occur if one is taken off a steroid too quickly.

Treatment: Topical

Treatment of atopic dermatitis will be basically the same as treatment for the other types of dermatitis to be discussed in this book. Therefore you should pay close attention to this section, as I will use it for reference.

'If it is wet, dry it. If it is dry, wet it' – that is an old saying often repeated in medical circles, but not by dermatologists who view their methods as much more sophisticated. It is a comment made by doctors in other specialities, usually internists (specialists in internal medicine) or surgeons who do not believe there is much to treating skin problems, nor to the field of dermatology in general.

Dermatologists cringe. Some fight back: 'What about that man who had simple dandruff? You thought he had a symptom of leprosy. It took a dermatologist to sort that out.' And so the struggle goes on.

However, every knowledgeable clinician, whether or not he or she is a skin doctor, knows that it takes a great deal of kindness, patience, knowledge and judicious use of medications to help an eczema sufferer.

There is a half-truth to the old saying, as there is to many old sayings. I can agree with the part that states 'If it is wet, dry it', but the second part about wetting a dry rash is not so good if taken literally. Dry skin and chronic rashes may get worse if they are frequently exposed to water or astringent compresses.

The weepy dermatitis of acute and subacute eczema does need to be dried before it can be effectively healed with topical preparations. The treatment of an acute or subacute dermatitis is fundamentally the same regardless of the cause, whether it is atopic dermatitis or a contact dermatitis.

1. *Acute and subacute dermatitis.* There are several ways a moist dermatitis can be dried. If it is not too weepy, the simplest method is to wash it well with a mild non-alkali soap such as Aveenobar or Aveenobar Oilated (both contain colloidal oatmeal which is soothing and mildly drying), Neutrogena or Oilatum.

A more weepy dermatitis can be dried with moist compresses of aluminium acetate (Burrows solution) or normal saline (0.9 per cent sodium chloride). The latter is a weak concentration of salt water which is analogous to the salty concentration of our body fluids. Normal saline can be used directly as it is. Aluminium acetate needs to be diluted 1:20 or 1:40, if the 1:20 dilution feels too strong after you apply the first compress. It should be diluted in tepid or cool water, not hot, as heat will make you itch. A 1:20 dilution is equivalent to one tablespoon of powder in a pint of water, while a 1:40 dilution is equal to one tablespoon of powder in one quart of water. Compresses should be applied for fifteen to twenty minutes, three times a day, to the oozing crusted areas. Hands and feet are more readily soaked in a basin of the solution, rather than compressed.

If the dermatitis covers extensive parts of your body, or is around the rectum or genitals, a fifteen-minute daily soak in an Aveeno Colloidal Oatmeal bath will be an effective drying method. Cornstarch baths do the same thing, and are cheaper. These baths also help relieve itching. If necessary, for additional relief, an oral antihistamine may be taken (see List 4, pages 50–51).

All the substances mentioned for drying a weepy dermatitis should be available from your chemist without a prescription. You can start this treatment right away while waiting to see the doctor. It not only dries the dermatitis, but also cleans away the crusts and surface bacteria. And it will not harm you.

If aluminium acetate or normal saline is not available at your chemist, you can dilute half a teaspoon of salt in a pint of lukewarm water and use that for a compress, or a hand and foot soak.

Potassium permanganate in a 1:8000 solution is frequently used in Britain as a soak for weepy hand and foot dermatitis. It is an old remedy, and a much stronger astringent than aluminium acetate or saline. Personally, I do not think it is that desirable, or necessary. If the powder or tablet is not dissolved well, the residue can cause burns. Also, potassium permanganate has a purple colour that will stain fabric and discolour finger- and toenails.

For a moist dermatitis, corticosteroid lotions, gels or sprays can be used. In addition to their steroid effect, each of these is also drying. The lotions spread nicely and penetrate well. They may produce stinging if the vehicle, or foundation substance for the steroid, contains propylene glycol. Sprays and gels may likewise cause stinging. The gels may be irritating if used too often and for too long a period. The physical force of the spray and occasionally the propellant substance carrying the steroid may produce stinging.

I think it is best to use a lotion, spray or gel on a moist dermatitis in flexures, creases or hairy areas of the body. Lotions are, usually, preferable because they spread well and sting less than gels or sprays. Certain fastidious or time-conscious patients might prefer the latter. On non-hairy areas, a corticosteroid cream is fine when combined with drying treatment, and is less likely to cause stinging.

The doctor can start you off with a cream at a potency which he or she thinks is most effective for you, depending on the severity and frequency of the dermatitis and how it has responded in the past to topical steroid treatment. Some dermatologists begin with a stronger cream, e.g. Betnovate, for a few days until the rash is under control, and then switch to a weaker steroid for the remainder of therapy. However, when the dermatitis is not too severe, it is best to begin with the least potent preparation at its least potent strength, since repeated and prolonged application of steroids can produce undesirable side-effects. A one per cent hydrocortisone cream ranked as mildly potent, or clobetasone butyrate 0.05 per cent (Eumovate) ranked as moderately potent, are good creams with which to begin treatment (see Chapter 10).

Any potentially sensitizing preparation should not be applied to weepy or broken skin. People with and without atopic dermatitis are more vulnerable when the skin barrier is disrupted. In this instance, the decreased sensitivity to skin allergens, as noted in atopic dermatitis, does not apply. Thus, topical medications containing the antibiotic neo-mycin, or an antihistamine, should not be used. Both are well-known potential sensitizers. An allergic contact derma-titis along with your weepy rash would be adding insult to injury. Therefore, be alert to combination medication, such as hydrocortisone and neomycin creams, and question the doctor about this if he or she should prescribe such a preparation.

If there is an infection when the skin is broken, it would be best to treat it with an internal antibiotic. Erythromycin, 250 mg four times a day, is a good choice, with rare side-effects or allergic reactions.

2. *Chronic dermatitis.* Relief from itching, lubrication and resolution of the dermatitis are the primary goals in treatment. To refresh your memory, the skin is involved with itchy, dry, scaly patches, whose skin surfaces show thickening and increased skin markings which resemble 'elephant hide' or the surface of lichen ('lichenified' is a medical adjective used to describe chronic dermatitis). The dermatitis may form thick lichenified plaques of 1 to 6 cm in diameter to involve various and extensive parts (primarily flexor), or one or two plaques may be the only problem. The following discussion gives information about treatment.

What you can do before the doctor's visit. Topical anti-itch medications are not very effective, although there are several on the market. Some of these – the topical antihistamines and anaesthetics – should not be used at all. After a period of use they cause allergic contact rashes. True, in atopic dermatitis your capacity for developing this reaction is diminished, but it is not non-existent. If your skin is scratched or cracked from dryness, you run a risk of developing contact allergies or irritations from medications that are known to cause this. So avoid antihistamines such as Anthical, Anthisan, Caladryl, Phenergan and RBC, and topical anaesthetics like Anethaine, Locan, Nestosyl, Solarcaine and Xylocaine. They have no place in eczema.

If you are determined to buy something for the itching (the medical name is pruritus), try one of the plain calamine creams, ointments or oily lotions. These may also be used in acute dermatitis. They will not be terribly effective and are messy on the skin, but they are harmless. A commonly used preparation is Eczederm Cream which contains about 2 per cent starch in an emollient base.

You can also take an antihistamine by mouth. It is unlikely

to cause skin sensitization, but remember that most internal antihistamines make you drowsy, so do not take them while driving, operating dangerous machinery, drinking, or with sedatives and tranquillizers (for various oral antihistamines, see List 4, pages 50–51).

However, you would be better off to take cool baths, avoid irritating clothing and soaps, or take fifteen-minute daily soaks in Aveeno Oilated, which contains a soothing protein fraction of oat, and apply liquid paraffin for dryness. Or a bath with another emollient bath preparation may restore enough oil and moisture to your skin to counteract some of your discomfort. When using bath oils be careful not to slip and fall. To minimize this risk you may want to avoid oil soaks and apply the oil directly to your damp skin, then pat off the excess with a towel.

Some emollient bath preparations are:

Alpha-Keri Bath
    Liquid paraffin: 91.7 per cent
    Oil-soluble fraction of wool fat: 3 per cent
Aveeno Oilated
    Oat (protein fraction): 40 per cent
    Liquid paraffin: 37 per cent
Balneum
    Soya oil: 84.75 per cent
Emulsiderm
    Liquid emulsion containing liquid paraffin: 25 per cent
    Isopropyl myristate: 25 per cent
    Benzalkonium chloride: 0.5 per cent (a disinfectant helpful when there is secondary bacterial infection; it is inactivated by soap)
Oilatum Emollient
    Acetylated wool alcohols: 5 per cent
    Liquid paraffin: 63.7 per cent

The use of nightly bath oils should be combined with two to three times daily applications of emollient creams or ointments to the dry rash. There are several of these preparations available (see List 1, pages 45–8). The ointments are heavy and greasier preparations, while the creams are lighter and work into the skin more easily. When used without bath oils both are best applied after your usual bath or wash, while the skin is still moist. If applied in this way, they will seal in the moisture and be more effective in rehydrating your skin.

Bath oils and topical emollients may be enough to clear up minor attacks of chronic dermatitis. In any case, this combined treatment should be a daily routine for your general dry skin condition.

Skin ointments that contain salicylic acid and coal tar have been used, historically, for the treatment of chronic eczemas. Another traditional substance is ichthammol. Preparations of these medications exist either alone or in combination with one of the others. Zinc oxide, which has a protective and mildly beneficial effect, is often included in the combination (see List 2, pages 49–50).

Salicylic acid is a keratolytic. That means it breaks down surface scale, and smoothes the plaques of chronic dermatitis. Concentrations of 2 per cent are used first, gradually being increased to 3 per cent or 6 per cent if necessary. This medication should not be used on broken skin where it may cause a contact dermatitis and, if used over large areas, may be absorbed in enough quantity through the skin to cause toxicity.

Ichthammol is a stronger topical than salicylic acid, but not as strong as coal tar. Again, it can cause skin irritation and should not be used on open skin.

Coal tar is the most active of these preparations. It has both anti-itch and keratolytic properties. It is an unpleasant substance to use, since it is messy, smelly and stains clothing. Also it can be a skin irritant, and should not be used on inflamed or broken skin. Other side-effects are acne-type eruptions at the site of application, and production of skin sensitivity to the sun.

If you want to use tar, it is best for thick scaly plaques. Occasionally a chronic eczema will clear with a tar preparation after a steroid cream has not been completely successful by itself. In general, tar is used infrequently for eczema these days. The primary use is in psoriasis, where it can be an effective treatment when combined with ultraviolet sun exposure. Its enhancement of sun sensitivity is put to good use here to cause involution of the psoriasis. (See List 2, pages 49–50, for the names of some salicylic acid, icthammol and coal tar preparations.)

Your doctor's approach. Corticosteroids have revolutionized the treatment of skin diseases and have made most of the older preparations once used for dermatitis almost obsolete. This group of drugs, known also by the abbreviated name steroids, are the first choice for today's doctors (see Chapter 10).

A wide range of topical steroids are now available with varying degrees of potency. They are put into groups according to potency, with IV indicating the mildest potency and I indicating the greatest potency.

A good medication with which to begin treatment in thicker, chronic dermatitis is a steroid of moderate potency. There are several in this group, such as Tridesilon, Eumovate, Haelan, Cloderm and Ultradil. They come as creams, ointments and lotions. An ointment gives more lubrication and penetrates better but is greasy. It is best used on very dry, thick areas. Lotions are best used in hairy areas, e.g. the scalp or in creases where greater drying is required. Gels would be used in the same places.

If the dermatitis shows resistance to the medication, or resolution is not progressing as quickly as is hoped, the effectiveness of the drug can be increased by covering the treated area with a clear plastic wrap for eight to twelve hours. Creams are best used with this type of occlusion, as the ointment gets gooey, and lotions are not used on chronic dermatitis in non-hairy regions. The plastic used for occlusion is the ordinary, household clear plastic wrap which is used to cover vegetables and other foods. When the area to be occluded is a limb, the plastic sheet can be simply wrapped round it and overlapped at the edge. It will adhere to itself. A strip of Sellotape on the overlapped edges, not on the skin, will secure it further. If the plastic wrap has to be cut as a square and taped over a plaque, hypoallergenic tape (Dermicel) should be used.

Hypoallergenic tape impregnated with steroid can be used in place of the occlusion and taped directly on to the thickened area to be treated. This method, of course, could never be used in a moist dermatitis, and should not be attempted. Steroid tape is a more expensive way of getting increased amounts of steroid into the dermatitis than is plastic occlusion. Therefore, it is recommended less often. The use of plastic occlusion is also decreasing as more potent steroid creams become available.

Plastic occlusion produces moisture and warmth and enhances the penetration of the steroid several-fold, and hence hastens the improvement of the problem. Occlusion also increases the possibility of side-effects from the steroids. These are thinning of the skin with fragility, increased formation of tiny blood vessels or capillaries, and a greater chance of skin infection. The same complications may occur if a steroid cream is used over too long a period. The more potent the cream, the greater its effect and, hence, the greater are the chances of side-effects. Therefore it is desirable to begin with a lower potency cream and work up if the lower dose does not work.

If large areas of the body are occluded or if a strong steroid cream is applied daily over a wide area, systemic absorption

41

can occur through the skin. The patient may experience internal effects of the steroid. The earliest change will be suppression of his or her own internal (endogenous) steroid secretion from the adrenal cortex. This can weaken the patient's resistance to infection and stress. Other side-effects can occur if the absorption through the skin continues (see Chapter 10).

Internal effects of topically applied steroids are infrequent, since large body areas are not involved in most patients and the medication will therefore be limited to small, specific regions. Nevertheless, the potential for systemic effects should be kept in mind.

Although most doctors use steroids to treat chronic dermatitis, some still like to dabble with the older remedies which are less costly than steroids. These doctors may recommend a salicylic acid, ichthammol or coal tar cream. Bufexamac is another non-steroid cream which may be used for mild chronic rashes. When it was first introduced there was hope that it might be an effective non-steroid alternative. But its activity is weak, and like the other non-steroid drugs it can irritate broken skin.

The doctor will also tell you to use a mild soap, to use emollients for your skin when the rash clears, and to put emollient bath additives into your water or onto your skin after bathing. In short, he will instruct you in good general skin care.

Hydroxyzine (Atarax) tablets are a relatively effective and frequent prescription for itching. The drug also has a tranquillizing effect which is helpful to someone with a severe itch. Antihistamines may be prescribed instead (see List 4, pages 50–51). Sometimes a tranquillizer such as Valium is given to the patient, and a sedative at night. These medications, if needed, may be prescribed at any of the three stages of dermatitis.

If the scalp is involved a steroid lotion will be prescribed.

Special shampoos that help eliminate scale should be used. Many of these are tar shampoos (see List 3, page 50). Pyrithione zinc shampoos (Zincon) are also good to use.

Thick plaques that do not respond fast enough are occasionally injected with a steroid solution. Triamcinolone acetonide (Adcortyl, Ledercort) in a concentration of 2.5 mg/ml is the preferred injectible. This intralesional injection has to be done carefully: 1 ml, a maximum of 2 ml for larger lesions, is all that should be injected, although some dermatologists say one can inject as much as 5 ml. Too much steroid deposited at one site will not only dissolve the plaque, but also the skin with its underlying fat. Instead of a plaque, you may end up with a dip in the skin. And the skin will be thin, shiny, brownish in colour with prominent small blood vessels. This defect will eventually correct itself, but it will take a long time. In the meantime, you will have an unsightly spot.

On the other hand the injection does work quickly, and the steroid preparation is such that it will stay at the site of the injection and not disperse throughout the body.

Treatment: General

The first thing you have to do is come to terms with your disease. You have to accept the fact that you have a hereditary predisposition to break out in the way you do when you are stressed or when your skin is irritated. Understand that the biochemical genetic fault or faults have yet to be discovered for atopic dermatitis. Since the origin is unknown, a cure cannot be attempted.

The disease is often chronic and variable. It comes and goes and can last for several years. Although it cannot be cured, it can be controlled. You will have trouble-free months and years between outbreaks, and you should have fewer and fewer eruptions as you get into middle age and older.

Stress is a definite trigger. Learn to relax, get away from

stressful situations. Get adequate rest and sleep. If you need counselling, talk to your doctor about a referral.

Remember, heat aggravates your rash. Do not get over-heated; be careful about excessive exertion in hot weather. Avoid extreme heat in general. Extreme cold can also irritate your skin.

Wear loose, comfortable clothing that allows air to circulate and keeps you cool. Fabrics next to the skin should be cotton. Avoid irritating material such as wool, nylon or satin. Also avoid contact with irritants in your work and at home. Wear gloves with a thin cotton glove as inner lining for protection when you do housework, work outdoors or with any solvents or chemicals.

Your skin is inherently dry, and dry skin is more susceptible to irritation and subsequently to a breaking out of the dermatitis. Therefore, you should get into a lifelong habit of taking care of your skin. Do not use harsh soaps. If your skin is extremely sensitive to bathing and even to non-alkali soap, wash only under the arms and in the genital areas daily. Wash the rest of the skin only when necessary.

When you bathe, use a bath oil (non-perfumed) in the bath water or directly on to your moist skin after a bath. If you put the oil into the bath, be careful not to slip (use a rubber mat). Cream your skin at least twice daily with one of the emollients.

Baths should be cool, never hot. A cold compress to an itchy area will often provide relief.

Be positive. Your rash will not kill or maim you. Don't become a social recluse. In time, the dermatitis will go away.

Systemic Steroids: When to Use Them, if at All
The two clear indications for the use of internal steroids are autosensitization with spreading of the rash, and generalized exfoliative dermatitis. In general, doctors do not like to use systemic steroids for chronic conditions because of the com-

plications that can occur from long-term exposure to them (see Chapter 10). There is no question that internal steroids will quickly clear the rash and make you comfortable. However, it may be difficult to get off them. When the dose is dropped, you may experience a 'rebound', which means the rash flares up again. This forces the doctor to increase the dose once more in order to control the rash. Sometimes the new controlling dose has to be even higher than the original dose. In the meantime, you continue to be exposed to a potent drug which is altering your body chemistry, with attendant side-effects.

The best and safest course is to control the dermatitis with topical steroids, since they have fewer internal effects.

However, if the dermatitis is creating a social or professional crisis in your life – you cannot get married with eczema all over your body, or you cannot give that speech while you are scratching – systemic steroids are in order. They can be given either by mouth for several days, or by weekly or biweekly intramuscular injection. There is better control over daily dosage if the drug is taken by mouth.

If you are under continuing emotional stress with constant exacerbations and itching, small daily or alternate-day doses will be helpful.

The following lists, and those on pp. 163–8, give medications useful in the treatment of many skin diseases discussed in this book. They should be a helpful source of information and will be referred to frequently. The majority of preparations in Lists 1–4 can be purchased over the counter; those in Lists 5 and 6 need a doctor's prescription.

LIST 1: EMOLLIENTS AND BARRIER PREPARATIONS

CREAMS

These either mix with water and are easily washed off, or

are oily and not readily washed off. They contain preservatives to counteract bacterial and fungal growth. At times, these preservatives might be sensitizers. Be alert to this if a rash occurs at the site of application.

Urea is incorporated into some creams. It is a hydrating agent, useful in dry, scaling dermatitis. It may also be used with corticosteroids to enhance their penetration.

Lanolin (hydrous wool fat) in emollients may sensitize the skin.

Other ingredients incorporated into creams are *menthol*, *camphor* and *phenol*. These have a mild anti-itch effect. *Calamine* and *zinc oxide* may also be used to enhance the effect.

Zinc and *titanium* additive have mild astringent benefits, but basically are used for protective preparations. Zinc preparations are primarily used in infantile eczema to protect the nappy area against urine.

Dimethicone and other silicones are water-repellent substances incorporated into creams to give protection against irritation from external substances and water. Chemists doubt whether these silicone creams are any better than the common zinc compounds. Furthermore, they have the potential to sensitize, especially already irritated skin. Actually, one could very easily do without these.

Some creams are:

Alcoderm
Aqueous Cream
Buffered Cream
Diprobase Cream
E45 Cream (contains lanolin)
Eczederm (contains calamine and starch)
Locobase
Masse' Breast Cream (nipple care and rashes)
Natuderm

Oilatum
Prehensol (in vanishing cream – detergent dermatitis)
Ultrabase
Vaseline Intensive Care (contains one per cent
  dimethicone)
Urea Creams (contain 10 per cent urea)
  Aquadrate (comes as ointment too)
  Calmurid
  Nutraplus

OINTMENTS

These are greasy preparations, not soluble in water, and more occlusive than creams. Since they are messy, the creams are more cosmetically acceptable. Modern formulations mix with water and fat, and may have a mild anti-inflammatory effect. Their occlusive properties on the skin's surface encourage hydration. Macrogols in these ointments produce the water solubility. This also means they can be washed off readily.

Ointments are beneficial in chronic dry dermatitis. Those that contain wool fat (lanolin) or wool alcohols (lanolin alchohols) may cause sensitivity in susceptible people.

Some ointments are:

Cetamacrogol Emulsifying Ointment
Emulsifying Ointment
Hydrous Ointment
Hydrous Wool Fat (lanolin)
Hydrous Wool Fat Ointment
Kamillosan Ointment (nappy rash, chapped hands)
Macrogol Ointment
Paraffin, White Solution (white petroleum jelly)
Paraffin, Yellow (yellow petroleum jelly)
Paraffin, Yellow Soft (yellow petroleum jelly)
Wool Alcohols Ointment

Diprobase Ointment
Locobase Ointment

BARRIER PREPARATIONS (CREAMS, OINTMENTS AND PASTES)
Dimethicone Cream (10 per cent dimethicone)
Titanium Dioxide Paste (pastes contain thickening substances such as kaolin, talc, also finely powdered zinc oxide; sometimes starch. The latter is not present in titanium dioxide. Titanium dioxide is used for nappy and urinary rashes, and as a sunscreen.)
Zinc Paste Compound (zinc oxide 25 per cent, starch 25 per cent in white soft paraffin)
Zinc Cream (contains 8 per cent wool fat [lanolin])
Zinc Ointment (15 per cent zinc oxide in simple ointment)
Zinc and Castor Oil Ointment (nappy and urinary rash)
Siopel (10 per cent dimethicone; nappy rash)
Sudocream (contains 4 per cent wool fat [lanolin]; primary ingredient: 15 per cent zinc oxide; urinary rash)
Thovaline Ointment (zinc oxide 20 per cent; urinary, nappy rash)
Vasogen (20 per cent dimethicone, 7.5 per cent zinc oxide; nappy, urinary rash, itchy anal area)

LOTIONS
These are water-soluble suspensions or solutions which have some cooling effect on the skin when contrasted to creams or ointment.
Some emollient lotions are:
Alcoderm
Emulsiderm
Keri Lotion (contains lanolin oil)
Lacticare lotion
Phisoderm lotion (contains lanolin)

LIST 2: SALICYLIC ACID, ICHTHAMMOL AND COAL TAR PREPARATIONS FOR PSORIASIS AND CHRONIC DERMATITIS

Antipeol Medico Ointment (ZnO, ichthammol, salicylic acid in urea)

Erytex CP Ointment (calamine 12.5 per cent, ZnO 10 per cent and salicylic acid 1.25 per cent)

Ichthammol Ointment (10 per cent ichthammol)

Zinc and Ichthammol Cream (5 per cent ichthammol, 10 per cent lanolin in zinc cream)

Zinc Paste and Ichthammol Bandage (for thick, crusted dermatitis)

Zinc Ichthopaste and Ichthaband (impregnated zinc paste and ichthammol bandage; very thick plaques)

Salicylic Acid Cream and Ointment (about 2.5 per cent salicylic acid)

COAL TAR PREPARATIONS (FOR THICK ECZEMAS; AVOID INFLAMED OR IRRITATED SKIN)

Alphosyl Cream (5 per cent coal tar extract, 2 per cent allantoin in vanishing cream)

Calamine and Coal Tar Ointment

Carbo-Dome Cream (10 per cent coal tar)

Clinitar Cream (1 per cent coal tar extract)

Coal Tar and Salicylic Acid Ointment

Coltapaste (impregnated zinc paste and coal tar bandage)

Pragmatar Ointment or Cream (4 per cent coal tar distillate, 3 per cent salicylic acid, 3 per cent precipitated sulphur)

Zinc and Coal Tar Paste

TAR BATH PREPARATION (FOR THICK, DRY ECZEMA ONLY)

Polytar Emollient

COAL TAR AND STEROID PREPARATIONS

Alphosyl HC Cream (0.5 per cent hydrocortisone added to it)

Carbo-Cor (hydrocortisone 0.25 per cent, coal tar solution 3 per cent)

Cor-tar-quin (2 per cent coal tar, 0.5 per cent hydrocortisone, 1 per cent of a hydroxyquinoline – latter for surface infection)

Tarcortin (5 per cent coal tar extract, 0.5 per cent hydrocortisone)

LIST 3: HELPFUL SHAMPOOS

Take care if scalp is scratched or has open sores; in which case these shampoos might cause stinging and burning.

Betadine Shampoo (when there are infected areas)

Ceanel Concentrate

Clinitar Shampoo

Genisol

Ionil T

Lenium Cream Shampoo (contains selenium sulphide 2.5 per cent)

Polytar Shampoo and Polytar Plus

Selsun

Synogist

T/Gel (2 per cent coal tar extract)

LIST 4: OVER-THE-COUNTER ORAL ANTIHISTAMINES FOR ITCH

Remember: they often cause drowsiness, and alcohol should not be taken, also avoid driving and operating machinery.

Actidil (triprolidine hydrochloride, 2.5 mg tablets)

Anthisan M & B (mepyramine maleate, 50 mg tablets)

Benadryl (diphenhydramine hydrochloride, 25 and 50 mg tablets)

Daneral S.A. (pheniramine maleate, 75 mg sustained-release tablets)

Dimotane (brompheniramine maleate, 4 mg tablets)

Histryl Spansule (diphenylpyraline hydrochloride, 5 mg sustained release)

Lergoban Sustained Release (diphenylpyraline hydrochloride, 5 mg)

Phenergan M & B (promethazine hydrochloride, 10 and 25 mg tablets)

COIN-SHAPED DERMATITIS

Another name for this eruption is 'discoid' dermatitis. The medical name – again resorting to the Latin – is *Nummular dermatitis*. 'Nummular' means 'circular' or 'coin-shaped', and refers to the appearance of the typical lesions. These are discrete circles or ovals with rather indistinct borders, about the size of a fifty-pence piece or smaller. They can combine to get larger if the disease worsens. Like all the eruptions in the dermatitis group, this one can be acute, subacute, or end up as a chronic dermatitis with thick, scaly, discrete areas of lichenification.

Initially, it begins as itchy tiny papules and vesicles which soon combine to form a red, moist, scaly patch, as the vesicles break from irritation, scratching or degeneration of the overlying skin. Secondary superficial infection is common and becomes an important contributing component.

Unlike atopic dermatitis, nummular eczema occurs on the extensor parts of the body – first appearing on the front of the legs, thighs and tops of the feet. The outside parts of the arms and tops of the hands may also be involved, as may the rest of the body, but this is less common.

Many skin doctors believe that nummular dermatitis is related to atopic dermatitis. This connection may seem clearer in children whose atopic lesions have a coin-shaped appearance. In adults, evidence for an association is ambiguous – many give no history of a preceding eczema. However, it is evident that there is a predisposition in some people to develop this dermatitis. Afflicted patients often have a skin that is drier than normal. Emotional stress is, also, an important factor in the initiation and progress of the disease.

The onset is abrupt, and the course is variable. It may quickly clear with treatment and that is the end of it. More commonly, it will persist with ups and downs over a period of a couple of years. When it does recur, it tends to appear at the original sites of involvement.

Treatment

Treatment is the same as that for dermatitis in general (see Atopic Dermatitis, pp. 20 ff.). The acute phase of the disease should be dried with mild soaps or compresses of an astringent solution like aluminium acetate. A hydrocortisone cream or lotion can then be applied.

In this dermatitis, the use of topical antibiotics is valuable. Neomycin can be used topically by itself with a companion corticosteroid preparation, or one of the neomycin-steroid combination creams can be prescribed. Neo-Cortef Cream or Ointment is an adequate starter (for discussion of these agents, see Chapter 10).

Terra-Cortril ointment, which contains 3 per cent oxytetracycline with one per cent hydrocortisone cream, may be substituted if you are sensitive to neomycin or there is concern that you might develop a sensitivity. Terra-Cortril does not cover as wide a spectrum of bacteria as neomycin, and bacteria at times become resistant to it.

When they do not wish to worry about the possibility of neomycin sensitization, some doctors may also prescribe Trimovate Cream (a combination of emovate steroid, nystatin and oxytetracycline). However, it contains nystatin, which is not a necessary medication in treatment of discoid dermatitis.

For chronic patches of nummular dermatitis, moderately potent or potent steroids will usually clear the rash.

An ointment salve is good to use, since it penetrates better than the cream, and helps to lubricate. Lubrication is an important part of treatment. The lesions are discrete and often confined to extremities, so ointments are less likely to make a mess of one's clothes.

Correction of the underlying skin dryness is important in the overall treatment. You should use bath oil in your bath and emollients on your skin, and make this a habit. Antihistamines, mild tranquillizers or sedatives may be needed to control itching.

Every attempt should be made to correct underlying anxiety and worry which may contribute to the chronic course.

Thick, resistant chronic plaques may be treated with one of the salicylic acid, coal tar preparations to dissolve the scales (see List 2, pages 49–50). This treatment should then be supplemented with topical steroids which may also be injected into extra stubborn lesions, if you are particularly anxious to rid yourself of a spot. Systemic steroids are rarely needed for this dermatitis.

What Else Can Look Like It?

The most likely condition to be confused with nummular dermatitis is Winter's Itch which I shall discuss next.

The basic problem in the latter is excessively dry skin. The confusion arises when this cracked dried skin develops a nummular-like eczema.

Ringworm may also resemble nummular dermatitis (see pp. 114–19). Both begin as oval, scaly pink or red lesions. Ringworm also starts as tiny blisters in its early stage and often affects the extremities. But ringworm does not itch, and the oval lesions spread peripherally, producing an arc of tiny blisters with clearing at the centre of the lesion. When the dermatologist does a scraping of the edge of the ringworm infection, he will be able to see fungal elements under the microscope. This will clinch the diagnosis, if there is clinical doubt.

Allergic contact dermatitis may at times be confused with nummular eczema. It also itches and its discrete lesions may look like the discrete lesions of discoid dermatitis. The difference is in distribution and a history of a contact exposure to the involved areas.

WINTER'S ITCH

Unlike the seven-year itch, winter's itch can be treated readily without any major disruptions in personal behaviour or psychology, for winter's itch is quite simply due to excessively dry skin.

Asteatotic (meaning without oil) dermatitis is a very apt description, and another term for it. Basically, the skin of the patient becomes dry because of a decrease in the fat or lipid layer.

As you age, body oil glands make less fatty substances, and the skin itself becomes thinner, drier and less capable of retaining moisture. This is a part of the normal ageing process, but in some people it is accentuated. They may inherently have drier skin, or they may have an underlying disease process that encourages skin dryness, or the skin can dry out from medications, the environment or certain habits, such as sitting before an electric heater when the weather is cold. The middle-aged and elderly, especially the latter, are most likely to develop winter dermatitis. Men are the most frequent sufferers.

A common site for its appearance is the extremities. To begin with, the skin is drier here than on other parts of the body and, furthermore, is more exposed to dryness from the elements.

The first sign is a dry and flaky skin. If this is neglected, the skin begins to crack. This fragmentation involves the very top, scaling layer called the stratum corneum (see Fig. 5, p. 15). It gets broken up into irregular dry areas with narrow, reddish fissures between them. A black and white photograph would resemble the parched cracked bottom of a clay bed. The superficial split patches of skin pull away from each other. Their edges curl up slightly, creating a flaky, dry fringe, while fissures between the patches are pink and shiny, denuded of their protective cover.

The fissures are breaks in the skin's protective barrier. They permit the skin to get more readily irritated and more readily infected. The dryness and irritation produce itching and consequent scratching further traumatizes the skin.

If you are unaware of the drying process, or how to correct it, you will continue to use harsh soaps, bathe too much or apply things to your skin which continue to dry and aggravate it. Sometimes, you may think that 'rubbing alcohol' is beneficial, because it feels cool and gives temporary relief from itch. But it is not. It is one of the worst things you could put on your skin, and will dry and crack it drastically, aggravating the problem.

The wind and low humidity of cold winter days dry skin. We all have experienced chapping because of a cold wind blowing against our cheeks or bare hands. If you are older and your skin is drier to begin with, this type of chapping is enhanced. Sleeping on an electric blanket to keep warm will further dry out your skin. All this predisposes you to the development of a winter dermatitis.

Medications such as diuretics, taken for heart disease or high blood pressure, will further dry your skin. Rubbing compounds, to relieve sore, aching muscles or pains of arthritis, will also dry your skin. Most of these contain drying lotions. Certain internal diseases such as hypothyroidism (low thyroid hormone secretion), diabetes or rarely a lymphoma (a cancer of the lymph glands) may produce asteatotic skin.

A dermatitis will develop if the dry skin is not treated, or an underlying cause corrected.

The skin now becomes more easily sensitized, irritated or infected. Soon the itchy, tiny blisters of acute dermatitis, with their red base, appear in the area of the fissures. They combine to form typical red, moist scaly patches.

The distribution will be on the extremities, commonly, and the dermatitic patches will begin as discrete ovals, often resembling nummular dermatitis. Indeed, there may be a point where it will be difficult to determine whether the rash is a nummular dermatitis or a dermatitis stemming from a dried-out skin.

The dermatitis can progress through its various stages (usually the acute or subacute) but, in practice, it is unusual to see a chronic stage of winter eczema. The itching and rash will drive you to see a doctor, who should make the right diagnosis and begin appropriate therapy.

Treatment

The prime treatment is directed at restoring oil and moisture to the skin. Therefore, elimination of harsh soap and any topical irritants is done. Bath oils and emollient creams are introduced as a part of daily routine. An ointment with urea added to its base will hydrate the skin also. This alone may be enough to clear up the problem.

Corticosteroid creams of mild to moderate potency should be adequate for treatment of the dermatitis. Ointments are preferred here, because they provide more lubrication.

Once your dry skin has improved and the rash has cleared, you will have to maintain emollient skin treatment in order to prevent a relapse. But by practising proper skin care and avoiding irritants you can prevent this dermatitis.

If the itchy dryness and dermatitis is persistent, an underlying factor should be sought. Blood tests which examine your white cells, red cells, thyroid level and blood sugar level should be done.

The effects of a diuretic can be counteracted with conscientious topical lubrication of the skin.

For itching which is driving you 'wild', antihistamines or Atarax (hydroxyzine hydrochloride) or a mild tranquillizer or sedative should give you relief while you are restoring your skin to good health.

HAND DERMATITIS

I remember a cartoon advertisement from my childhood, showing a young housewife in terrible distress. Her eyes were drawn downwards and there were deep vertical lines between her brows. She held her poor hands limply in front of her; they were coloured red with wavy lines indicating heat coming from them. 'Do your hands feel like lobster claws?', ran the ad. 'Has romance gone out of your life? Then try —.' I forget what it was that the woman was supposed to try, but whatever it was it was miraculous. The last drawing showed her cuddling up to a husband who adoringly fondled her hands.

That was my first introduction to 'housewife's eczema' or 'washerwoman's eczema'. At the time, I was merely amused and .perplexed. I thought the red hands were advertising

57

hype. I had never seen a woman with that kind of problem. After all, my mother did a great amount of housework and she never had trouble with her hands. Since then I have come to realize that many women and men are bedevilled with hand dermatitis, and that washing liquids and soaps are not always the causative agents. Furthermore, it takes more than a simple hand cream to resolve the condition.

The general term 'hand dermatitis' encompasses any itchy, dermatitic condition of the hands, regardless of cause. This skin problem falls into two groups: hand rashes that occur from an external cause, and those that are secondary to some endogenous or internal source. In this chapter, we shall primarily concern ourselves with the latter, but I would like to mention a few things about the former.

External Hand Dermatitis
This is a contact dermatitis, due to repeated contact with an irritating or allergy-producing substance. Substances such as strong soaps, detergents, solvents are irritating and will cause itching, redness and cracking of the hands in most people (see Contributing Factors, pp. 62–3). However, if you have atopic dermatitis, your skin becomes more easily irritated and therefore is more apt to develop an irritant contact dermatitis. Conversely, an irritation of the hands can trigger an atopic dermatitis of the hands.

Certain substances will cause allergies of the hands in susceptible individuals. This will present as blisters, then as moist, oozing patches – the typical picture of acute or subacute dermatitis. Sometimes it will be hard to distinguish this from internal hand dermatitis to which the remainder of this section is devoted. For relevant information about external hand dermatitis, see Chapter 3.

Internal (Endogenous) Hand Dermatitis
The two medical names for this – dyshidrotic eczema or

dyshidrosis and *pompholyx* – are hang-overs from our Latin-naming predecessors. 'Dyshidrotic' means that there is an abnormality in sweat gland function. At one time, this was considered the causative factor, and the blisters or 'bubbles' which characterize the rash were thought to be sweat gland secretions. This has proved to be false. The blisters are full of body fluid, as in any dermatitis. 'Pompholyx' is a descriptive term, describing the 'bubble' appearance of the dermatitis. The word serves no useful purpose. Actually, both words are not only hard to pronounce, but archaic and misleading. They are also barriers to communication.

Doctors who are not dermatologists may not understand what is meant by these terms, not to mention the poor patient. After being told he or she has dyshidrotic eczema or pompholyx, it is likely the patient will leave the dermatologist's surgery believing he is afflicted with a bizarre, exotic malady. Nevertheless, dermatologists are stuck with these terms. Dyshidrotic eczema (read dermatitis) or dyshidrosis, in particular, are still used to identify a hand rash as being specifically from an internal source, rather than from a contact dermatitis.

Internal hand dermatitis occurs most often in children and adults to middle age. It seems to be more prevalent in the summer. Although there is no detectable pathological abnormality of the sweat gland, increased sweating of the hands is sometimes present. The precise significance of this is unknown.

A sudden eruption of small, itchy tense vesicles (blisters), 1 to 2 mm in size, heralds the onset of the rash. The skin under and around the vesicles is often lacking in redness, a somewhat different finding from other eczemas. This, plus the tenseness of the vesicles and their resorption without rupture, is undoubtedly due to the thick stratum corneum which is present on the palms. This thick topmost layer of skin physically prevents the blister from breaking, and also obscures the redness that reflects the inflammation accompanying the vesicles (see Fig. 7).

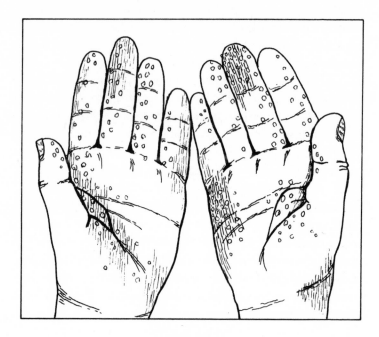

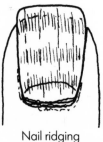

Nail ridging

Fig. 7 Hand Dermatitis – Typical Appearance of the Internal Type (also known as pompholyx or dyshidrotic eczema). Tiny, deep-seated blisters arise on the sides of the fingers and on the palms. These soon evolve into oozing or scaly red patches. Nails are often involved with ridging, mainly when there is a dermatitis right around them.

Scaling, dryness and increased skin lines are present in the chronic stage.

The vesicles have a very typical distribution which helps distinguish this from other hand rashes. The vesicles break out along the sides of the fingers and on the palms, often as a cluster in the middle of the palm. Involvement of the top of the hand or fingers does not occur usually, but does in allergic contact dermatitis.

The feet, which are physiologically analogous to the hands, may also break out. This eruption usually is not as marked and is often overlooked. However, in children, the dermatitis might present primarily as a foot problem.

Following blister eruption, scaling occurs. Some of the vesicles break as a result of scratching and some work their way to the very surface. In severe eruptions, vesicles may combine to form large blisters called bullae. These may be a centimetre in size.

The dermatitis usually affects both hands and is symmetrical. Like most of the dermatitides (plural of dermatitis), it has a variable course. It may last months, perhaps years, with periodic remissions and recurrences, or the duration can be short and self-limited.

Infections can complicate the problem, when the blisters coalesce or break to form weepy, crusted areas. Bacterial as well as yeast (candidal) infections can occur. The latter thrive in finger webs, where there is warmth and continuing moisture.

Also in an acute and subacute hand dermatitis, there is a greater chance for development of a secondary contact dermatitis – either of an irritant or allergic variety. This complicates things enormously, and makes evaluation difficult and the hand dermatitis hard to treat.

How to diagnose

By itself, an irritant contact dermatitis can be identified from dyshidrosis by its chapped appearance and the history of contact. A blistery allergic hand dermatitis, however, is harder to differentiate from dyshidrotic dermatitis. At times, it may be impossible to do so. The following factors help to make a distinction. A history of contact to an allergen is naturally valuable. Clinically, contact dermatitis, whether of irritant or allergic origin, tends to affect the tops of the hands, while dyshidrotic dermatitis is a disease of the palms and sides of the fingers. However, there are contactants that can involve these latter areas too (see Chapter 3). Patch tests to the allergen should be of great help in making the distinction.

Fungus infections in the acute stage may cause blisters on the palms, but this usually is self-limited. If it does progress, it will go into a chronic, scaling phase. A fungus infection of the hands is typically confined to one hand. A scraping of the involved skin will usually reveal fungal elements under the microscope, and a fungal culture will grow the organism.

These fungus infections are not yeast infections, but are infections called tinea, caused by organisms with long names like Trichophyton and Microsporum. They are common: athlete's foot is caused by them. An acute fungus infection of the feet may cause a secondary self-sensitization (autosensitization) blistery eruption of the palmar side of the hands. This should not be hard to diagnose, since the primary foot problem is usually apparent.

Contributing factors

So many factors may contribute to the cause of hand dermatitis that it is difficult to determine which one is pre-eminent.

The individual may have a predisposition to develop the eruption. It may be his or her weak target organ for continuing medical problems. Just as someone else might get an ulcer or high blood pressure when under stress, a person with this tendency will get hand eczema. You may be one of these people.

There are doctors who think hand dermatitis is a localized form of atopic dermatitis. This is hard to prove or disprove.

The rash may occur in atopic individuals or it may not. Many people with hand dermatitis give no history of atopic rashes, hay fever, asthma or hives – either for themselves or their families.

However, it is clear that hand dermatitis is a barometer of stress; anxiety will precipitate it and chronic anxiety will keep it going.

Irritating substances of various kinds can also trigger an internal hand rash. Once a rash develops, whether from initial stress or irritation, the irritants, along with continuing stress, will keep the dermatitis active.

Our hands are in contact with many things during the course of a day's work. The most common ones are soaps and detergents. In the kitchen, many foods and food juices can irritate the hands. Some of these are garlic, onion, tomato, spinach, citrus fruit, radish, parsnip, cheese.

Certain plant saps can irritate. Gloves should be worn when you garden.

Constant exposure to fluids or soaps causes maceration and defatting of the skin which leads to irritation and an eruption. In addition to housewives, bar-tenders, food handlers, doctors, dentists and chefs are at risk. Of course, if you work with solvents on your job, you are at high risk for irritation.

Treatment

The first step is to protect the hands: avoid irritants. Substitute non-alkali soaps, i.e. Basis, Neutrogena, Oilatum, for regular soaps. While washing dishes or clothes, wear gloves (plastic or rubber ones with a thin inner cotton glove). Of course, in the acute, oozing stage, you cannot wear gloves, but you should avoid all irritants and concentrate your energies on getting better.

Stress should be avoided. It may be advisable to keep away from work for a few days until the acute phase is brought under control. A short course of oral steroids for about five days, or an intramuscular injection of a corticosteroid may be needed to bring a swollen, badly inflamed dermatitis quickly under control. This will minimize the days that you will be handicapped.

Again, antihistamines or mild tranquillizers may be prescribed if you need them.

For infection, systemic antibiotics should be given. Topical antibiotics are not effective here. When the infection involves yeast organisms, topicals have to be used. Nystaform-HC or Terra-Cortril Nystatin, each of which contains 100,000 units of the anti-yeast drug nystatin with mild hydrocortisone, can be used. Trimovate is preferred by some doctors.

An oral drug is being used for resistant, chronic yeast infections of the nails and skin – this is Ketoconazole. However, it has side effects: liver toxicity has been reported. It has no place in the treatment of superficial candidal infections of a hand dermatitis. The available topicals, combined with hand soaks in aluminium acetate solution, 1:20 dilution, are adequate.

The acute dermatitis needs drying and debridement (clearing away) of crusts. As already mentioned, the aluminium acetate solution is valuable for that. A good time to apply corticosteroid creams is after soaking or at night. The doctor will probably start you off on a moderately potent steroid like Ultradil, and go to a stronger one, e.g. Betnovate, if there is little improvement.

Chronic dermatitis can be treated with a steroid ointment at night plus cortisone cream during the day. If the dermatitis is slow to respond, a steroid cream can be applied at night under occlusion, using a clear plastic 'baggie' or clear plastic glove. During the day emollient creams can be used to supplement the steroid applications, and should be in common use once the dermatitis clears.

When the dermatitis has healed or is into a chronic phase you can start wearing protective gloves. However, rubber or plastic gloves should not be worn by themselves. Hands sweat and the sweat inside the glove can be an irritant, and also cause maceration and further predispose the hands to sensitization to the rubber or plastic chemicals.

A routine I like for wearing protective gloves is as follows: make sure the hands are clean. Powder them lightly with a talc dusting powder that contains about 10 per cent starch – baby powder is suitable, too. Then don thin cotton gloves which can be purchased at cosmetic counters or a chemist's. These function as a protective lining against the rubber or plastic glove, while the talc picks up moisture from sweating. Lastly put on your plastic or rubber gloves. Wash dishes or clothes in lukewarm water. This will minimize the heat getting to your hands and lessen itching and sweating. When the cotton gloves get soiled, they can be washed or thrown away. With this method, your hands are not irritated with sweat or by contact with the outer gloves.

A *last word:* In a hand dermatitis, fingernails are often involved too. This happens when the rash involves the skin at the base of the nails. The inflammation will affect the cells forming the nail, since the nail grows from its base beneath the skin. The changes will commonly show up as ridging of the nail. The process can be aborted by applying steroid lotion or cream at the base and around the nail. In any case, damage is not permanent and healthy nails will be formed once the dermatitis clears.

DERMATITIS FROM VARICOSE VEINS

The lower part of the leg, just above the inner ankle area, is the most susceptible to varicose vein dermatitis or stasis dermatitis. Indeed, stasis is a major factor in causing this dermatitis.

Varicose veins have a hereditary background – someone in your family has probably been afflicted at some time. Women have them more commonly than men, and they often appear in pregnancy.

In contrast to arteries, venous walls are normally thin with scant contractile fibres. In varicose veins, you inherit weaker walls than is usual, and also weak valves. Thus, prolonged standing or any activity that produces increased pressure on the lower limbs will result in dilated, often tortuous (varicose) veins, and the valves which keep blood from flowing backward become incompetent. This may happen because of the widening of the vein wall, which prevents the valves from closing properly, or from a defect in the valves themselves.

The venous system is a relatively inert network. It depends on muscular movement and bodily activity to help propel the blood back to the heart. Activity is important. A person who is inactive, who does a great deal of immobile standing or sitting with the legs dependent, is at higher risk for development of varicose veins. The risk is greater when there is a familial predisposition.

The increased pressure and blood stagnation in the veins affect the entire dependent venous system down to the tiniest, microscopic vessel – the capillary. This is a one-celled structure with a thin lining. Capillaries exist throughout the body, but here we are concerned with skin capillaries. Increased pressure causes damage to the capillary lining and permits blood cells as well as protein rich blood fluids (serum) to escape into the skin. The red cells have no place to go, since they cannot re-enter the circulation. Therefore they are broken down in the skin into their biochemical iron component – a substance called haemosiderin. This sits in the skin causing a brownish discolouration. The extra body fluid in the tissues will appear as ankle swelling or oedema. It will be worse at night after you have been on your feet all day. In the morning it will be lessened or gone, as the pressure on your veins will have been relieved by bed rest. The oedema can be resorbed back into the body through the lymphatic system and intact capillaries while the red cells cannot.

If varicose veins are severe, or if there has been a deep vein thrombosis which blocks deep vein circulation, the skin changes will be much worse. The oedema will not be resorbed as well during the night. Some will remain in the tissue, leading to eventual scarring. The lower layer of skin, the dermis, will become toughened and still thicker than normal because of increased fluid. And the top layer, the epidermis, will have a thin shiny look with patches of scaling. The colour will be brownish-red, from the haemosiderin deposits and from the increased blood in dilated skin capillaries.

These changes have naturally damaged the skin. Itching will often be an accompanying symptom. If you scratch, you damage the skin further and set up a situation for infection.

This fragile skin is prone to skin irritation and allergic skin sensitization. You have to be careful about what you put on it: never any liniments or anything with rubbing alcohol (isopropyl alcohol) in it.

The damaged oedematous skin will crack on its own. Superficial infection and irritation then occur with an outbreak of an acute, weepy dermatitis. Thus stasis dermatitis begins.

It may clear, only to recur and so on. Like other dermatitis it may have a chronic scaly stage, but because of the accompanying oedema and tendency for fissuring of the skin, the dermatitis is, usually, subacute or acute.

An ulcer may develop, more often when the process is advanced or neglected. The ulcer may follow trauma – hitting your leg against something. Picking and scratching may also start it. The ulcer is characteristically right above the inner ankle area, often overlying an incompetent deeper vein. The location is so typical that an ulcer elsewhere on the leg usually points to another cause. The ulcer complicates the problem. It is a source of infection. Fluids oozing from it aggravate adjacent skin and further contribute to dermatitis.

An infection within the dermis of the skin may occur extending from an ulcer bed, or from a superficial infection in the stasis dermatitis itself. Systemic antibiotics and tepid compresses are in order.

Treatment

An ounce of prevention is worth a pound of cure. This old truism is no more true than here. If you have a tendency for varicose veins, take measures to prevent or impede their occurrence.

Exercise is important. You do not have to jog or do aerobics. A brisk thirty to sixty minute walk in the morning and evening is an excellent way to get your body moving, and will not damage your joints. Wear sensible shoes on your walks.

Keep moving. Do not stand without moving for longer than fifteen minutes. If you have to sit for long periods of time, this is not good either. Rest your feet on a small hassock or stool against which you can push and flex your feet. This contracts your calf muscles and stimulates venous flow. If you are at work or in a place where this is not possible, get up and move around every forty-five to sixty minutes. In the meantime, flex your feet and move your legs. Just because you are sitting or standing, you do not have to be immobilized. Elevate your feet. Rest them on a chair or stool about two or three inches above the horizontal plane of your body. This will drain blood and fluid away from the lower legs and into the general circulation. Do this for fifteen minutes two or three times a day. You can also elevate the foot of your bed a couple of inches with coasters or other means. This will relieve pressure from your legs and improve the oedema more rapidly.

Wear loose comfortable clothing. Do not wear anything that constricts your waist, your thighs or your legs. Tight belts, tight pants, girdles and garters are out. Too many times, I have seen older women, often overweight, come in for treatment of a stasis dermatitis with an elastic garter digging into the skin beneath their knees. This is like wearing a tourniquet and does nothing but hamper circulation and worsen the problem.

Support-hose are helpful during the day, especially if you have to do a lot of standing, or are a pregnant woman on her feet a lot. A word of caution: support-hose should fit properly. There should be a proper distribution of pressure from the ankle area to the thigh. The hose should not have a tourniquet effect on any part of your limb. Elastic bandages may be used instead of support hose. Men are more apt to wear them, since they can be hidden under trousers. For information about proper support-hose and the correct way to wrap on elastic bandages, you should consult your doctor or a knowledgeable nurse.

Lose weight if you are overweight. Obesity contributes to venous stasis and all the attendant problems. A typical patient with the chronic condition of stasis dermatitis and an accompanying ulcer is usually overweight.

When the dermatitis sets in

Again treatment is similar to that for other acute or subacute dermatitides. Often there is an attendant skin infection. This may be superficial and will clear with compresses. If not, systemic antibiotics will be prescribed. Erythromycin is a drug of choice in many uncomplicated skin infections. Topical anti-infectives such as the antibiotic neomycin or the anti-infective hydroxyquinoline, should be used with caution or not at all. The dermatitic skin here is at high risk for sensitization by these known sensitizers.

Soothing steroid creams or ointments of moderate to mild

potency should be applied topically, and are effective (see Chapter 10).

Coal tar and salicylic acid preparations have no place in the treatment of stasis dermatitis. Both these substances can be irritants, and coal tar is a strong sensitizer for broken and damaged skin.

An *ulcer* will need compressing with normal saline or aluminium acetate solution. First, it may need to be de-brided by the doctor (this means clearing away the ulcer's crust, scales and pus – usually mechanically by trimming or washing). Most doctors will have their own preferred way of treating ulcers, but compressing should be a basic procedure. A 3 per cent hydrogen peroxide solution may be used to clean the ulcer after the compresses. Infection will often be present and require systemic antibiotics. At the same time the dermatitis accompanying the ulcer will be treated with soothing steroid creams of mild to moderate potency. The milder the effective potency, the better. Over a period of time steroids thin the tissue, and in this case the skin is already atrophic. The doctor can add insult to injury if he or she is not careful.

Ulcers will take time to heal. Fortunately, most of them are smaller than a fifty-pence piece. Their progress should be monitored by the doctor. After healing the patient should wear support hose or bandages, and take very good care of the skin. Use non-irritating emollients (those without lanolin are preferable) and avoid trauma of any kind.

When to consult the vascular surgeon?

Stasis dermatitis is obviously not just a skin problem, but an end result of an underlying problem. Therefore, a surgeon should be seen early, as soon as you detect a varicose problem. It is possible that a stasis problem can be aborted by judicious varicose vein surgery.

Some ulcers will not heal easily with topical treatment,

and may need a surgical consultation with eventual skin grafting to the ulcer.

If you have never seen a vascular surgeon, ask for a consultation during the treatment for your stasis dermatitis. He may not be able to do anything definitive, but you should have a vascular opinion for a problem that is basically vascular.

VARIANTS

Certain localized eczemas exist in predisposed individuals. They soon evolve into chronic forms that may persist for years with periodic limited improvement. There may be a psychological overlay to these conditions. Anxiety may initiate them, or the habitual rash may be an expression of some psychological need. In the latter, the rash itself fulfils a psychic gratification. Cure may be difficult, until the patient finds substitute emotional gratification in his or her personal life, or undergoes appropriate psychotherapy.

Fortunately, these rashes are not serious and do not compromise a person's life very much. But they are itchy nuisances.

There are dermatologists who think these eczemas are localized manifestations of atopic dermatitis. There is no definite proof for this, although atopic dermatitis may exist for a time, confined to one area. Then you will have the other signs of atopic dermatitis too. Conversely, an atopic dermatitis occurring with a pre-existing local ezcema is very unusual.

Lichen Simplex Chronicus or Simple, Chronic, Lichen-Appearing Dermatitis
When I was in medical school, a dermatology professor would go on at great length about *lichen simplex chronicus*

71

and the *locus minoris resistentiae*. He would utter the words in a stentorian tone, with great emphasis and curling of his tongue around the Latin phrase. Periodically he would pounce. His hand went straight out pointing at me, while his eyes focused on someone to the other side of the room. The man was cross-eyed. Terror-ridden students never knew whether he meant to question the student pinned at the end of his finger, or the one riveted by his eyes. Invariably, two would stand up at once. He would ignore the one on which his eyes seemed to focus, and continue to jab his hand at the other one. He liked to pick on women. I would rise, quaking, my head swimming with Latin phrases, and would mumble something about the 'site of least resistance', and so on. He would say 'Sit down', and that would be the end of it.

Ever since, the phrases *lichen simplex chronicus* and *locus minoris resistentiae* have been implanted in my brain. He was telling us that a simple chronic rash, once begun, would continue to recur in the same spot which was the site of least resistance or *locus minoris resistentiae*. He did not explain what the biochemical and immunological conditions were that encouraged this. He did not know that, nor, for that matter, do we know that today.

In *lichen simplex chronicus*, abbreviated as LSC, the rash always comes back in the same spot.

It begins with a nervous scratching or rubbing of the skin which creates more itching and more scratching until the skin breaks out into small red papules and vesicles that combine to form a scaly patch of dermatitis. The habitual scratching will continue, especially when you are worried, anxious and under stress at work or at home. At times there are pleasurable sensations involved in the itching and scratching which keep the cycle going. The rash will soon evolve to a chronic stage to become a thick plaque, about 3 to 4 cm in size, with increased skin markings (lichen-like) and a dry scale. A tan discolouration is present since the inflammation and irritation cause the pigment-forming cells to discharge pigment into the dermal layer of the skin. This produces the colour. All these changes are reversible with treatment, but the pigmentation may take a long time to resolve, and may persist long after the rash has gone.

The dermatitis occurs as a single plaque and is well-localized. It develops more often in middle-aged women, usually on the nape of the neck. Other characteristic locations in both men and women are the outer ankle areas, the small of the back, side of the neck, forearms, navel area, the palm and the genital area (scrotum and vulva).

Severe itching is often described as the trigger that starts the cycle. It is not clear why the itching is confined to a certain area, nor what is the psychological benefit of this particular spot to the patient. The itching can provoke scratching to the point of pain. Women often use a comb to scratch the backs of their necks. Nail files, pumice stones – all sorts of things may be used for scratching. Men may sit in front of a television watching a soccer match, and work on their rash.

Treatment

Stop scratching and it will go away. If you can be persuaded to do that, you are lucky. The dermatitis will not return once it has cleared. But if you cannot do that, and you are in the majority, the dermatitis fulfils some emotional need and will continue to linger.

Topical treatment is usually all that is needed. Occasionally, you might need an antihistamine or mild tranquillizer. But a cold compress to the dermatitis will relieve itching too.

The salicylic acid/coal tar creams (see List 2, pages 49–50) may be used here to dissolve the surface scale and permit better penetration of a steroid cream. Again, the skin surface should be intact, if the former creams are to be used.

Since the plaque is thick, potent or very potent topical steroids can also be applied at night under plastic occlusion.

Thick resistant dermatitis may be an indication for intralesional steroid injections. Among the eczemas, LSC is the condition most frequently chosen for injection. The doctor should be careful not to inject too much into one spot at one time. If he or she does, there is the danger of atrophy of skin and underlying fat.

Steroid treatment clears the dermatitis but does not cure it. That seems to depend on resolving contributory psychological factors.

Breast Eczema

In women, the nipple or areola (the brown area surrounding the nipple) may develop a dermatitis. Itching and scratching in susceptible people aggravates this. Rough bras and those containing elastic may irritate or sensitize respectively, and should not be worn. Cotton bras with a soft, smooth cup are the best.

Avoid use of harsh soaps or topical preparations that might irritate (antihistamines, neomycin, coal tar, for example). A mild soap (Aveeno bar, Neutrogena) should be substituted. A soothing steroid cream or ointment is specific treatment. The nipple may be fissured and scaly. Hydrocortisone ointment is helpful here.

Nursing mothers, who have tendencies for eczema, may also develop a dermatitis of the nipple area. Masse' Breast Cream may be used for pre- and post-nursing nipple care.

A certain breast cancer, called Paget's Disease, begins with a dermatitis-type eruption of the nipple or areola. This is an uncommon entity, but a serious one. Topical treatment will clear eczemas but not the cancerous Paget's Disease. A breast dermatitis of more than a week's duration should be checked by a doctor. If the rash is unresponsive to treatment, it should be biopsied.

Dermatitis of the Genital and Anal Areas

Because of the location, a dermatitis here is primarily moist and subject to secondary infection. This area is also more prone to skin sensitization, more so when it is irritated.

Occlusive clothing, sweating, rubbing of skin surfaces, obesity, vaginal and anal discharges all contribute to the problem. Scratching further damages the skin. The macerated skin will often develop yeast infections (candidiasis), as well as bacterial infections. If the candidiasis is recurrent or persistent, you should be examined for underlying diabetes, since yeast infections are common with this disease.

Treatment

Comfortable, loose clothing should be worn. Avoid tight pants, rough fabrics. Next to the skin, cottons are preferred. Fabrics that have been treated to be crease-resistant and new polyesters should be washed first before they are worn. If' washing detergents aggravate, it may be necessary to double-rinse clothes.

It is important to keep the area dry. This can be done by washing three or four times daily with mild soaps, if the problem is minor. Sitz baths or compresses using aluminium acetate solution, 1:20 dilution, or normal saline are useful in acute problems. The washes or soaks should be followed with a steroid and anti-infective lotion, spray or cream.

Since bacteria and yeast often complicate this dermatitis, the initial preparation should contain an anti-fungal and anti-bacterial component. Once the dermatitis is under control, a plain steroid preparation can be used. To begin, a hydrocortisone, nystatin (anti-yeast) and oxytetracycline (anti-bacterial) cream may be used. (See List 5, pages 163–5.) The latter also comes as an ointment and spray without the nystatin. If bacterial infection is not a major problem, hydrocortisone/nystatin creams, lotions and ointments are available. Conversely, there are hydrocortisone/neomycin preparations to be used when yeast infection is not a concern. As mentioned before, neomycin on broken skin can be a sensitizer. In most cases it is not, or it would not be prescribed. Nevertheless, it is something to keep in mind.

When the area has been adequately dried, talc powders will help pick up moisture and continue to promote drying. Their use is beneficial in creases. Dusting powders with starch in them are the most helpful.

Barrier creams to protect against irritation from discharges may be used when the dermatitis has improved. These can be messy and are best applied at night. Those without dimethicone, which can sensitize, are preferable. Zinc cream and ointment are examples. A plain ointment or an ointment-based preparation will provide a good acceptable protective skin layer.

The psychosexual significance of some genital and anal eczemas makes them difficult to cure. Psychotherapy would be helpful here, but many patients because of embarrassment or denial will not seek this care. It is important for such patients to find a supportive person with whom they can discuss their problems. A kindly doctor, a counsellor, an understanding friend or family member can be helpful.

Dermatitis of the Outer Ear

This occurs behind the ear, inside the ear canal or on the ear lobe. The eruption may be a residual of atopic dermatitis or occur concurrently with it. Often there is no evident association.

Nervousness triggers the rash behind the ear and on the ear lobe. Other factors are also important when the ear canal is involved.

The outer ear canal is a blind passage into which ear wax and skin cells are normally shed. When itching develops, the tendency is to scratch – usually hard. Fingernails, hair pins, match sticks are some of the unsavoury objects that are used.

These not only damage the skin (at worst they even puncture an ear drum) but substances coating these objects may sensitize the skin. Nail polish on fingernails, nickel on hair pins and chromates on matches are culprits. A dermatitis will develop either from scratching, secondary infection or sensitization.

Drainage does not occur easily from a dead-end tortuous ear canal. Eczema fluid and cellular debris are good breeding grounds for opportunistic bacteria and fungi that normally reside in the ear canal without causing problems. This infection complicates the problem further.

Treatment

The ear canal needs to be dried and the infection treated if the rash is to improve.

A Q-tip dipped in normal saline (0.9 per cent sodium chloride), aluminium acetate (1:40 dilution), or 3 per cent hydrogen peroxide gently inserted with the cotton end fluffed and pulled out for greater absorbency, will dry the ear. This should be done three times daily. The drying solutions may be put into the ear by dropper, then gently absorbed with a cotton swab.

Combination steroid/anti-infective ear drops or lotions should clear the remainder of the ear canal problem.

The dermatitis on the outside of the ear can be treated with steroid creams or ointments.

The ear lobe, of course, should never be pierced while there is an existent rash. Even in the best of hands, pierced ears can get infected. Shortly after the procedure, twelve to forty-eight hours, redness and oozing occurs at the pierced site. The infected drainage irritates the surrounding skin and ear lobe and can additionally trigger an eczema in predisposed patients. Infective eczematoid dermatitis is the name given to this type of rash. As long as the earring is in place, the infection will not clear. Nickel in cosmetic jewellery can sensitize the damaged skin and add to the problem.

First, the earring must be removed. The area should be cleansed with a mild soap or one of the astringent drying solutions. A steroid/antibiotic cream is then applied. Occasionally, systemic antibiotics may be needed.

The pierced canal will grow over. You will be left with a tiny scar. Sometimes you may feel small cysts within the ear lobe at the pierced site. These may occur even when the ear does not get infected. These should be left alone and not manipulated. They tend to go away spontaneously.

Neurodermatitis

At one time, any patient who developed a rash when he or she was under stress was said to have neurodermatitis, a rash due to nerves. This soon became a catch-all term to cover any sudden itchy eruptions for which there was no apparent cause. Many of these rashes did have specific origins, but doctors did not know what they were, so they blamed them on nervous tension.

Today the term is not used very much. We try to give specific diagnoses. Occasionally, an older doctor accustomed to the traditional term will call a nummular dermatitis or atopic dermatitis a 'neurodermatitis'. Sometimes, a younger doctor, in desperation, not knowing what else to diagnose, will call something a 'neurodermatitis'.

Medical technology and research are providing information about biochemical processes that are factors in causing dermatitis. No longer can we say a dermatitis is just due to nerves. It is much more complex than that. True, anxiety and emotional stress can trigger a dermatitis and keep it active. But the patient has to have a genetic tendency for developing dermatitis under stress. Investigation of this 'tendency' will ultimately give us the specific cause or causes of a dermatitis. That knowledge will lead us to prevention and finally to cure.

Chapter Three

EXTERNAL GROUP (What You Touch, or What Touches You)

CONTACT DERMATITIS

Contact dermatitis is common. One out of ten patients coming to a skin clinic suffers from it. We are in contact with so many potentially noxious substances in our environment that it is surprising the incidence is not higher.

Two types of contact dermatitis exist: irritant and allergic. The latter resembles eczema and will primarily concern us. But something has to be said about irritant contact dermatitis because it is so prevalent. Your typical chapped red hands are an example.

Photosensitivity dermatitis, which requires the sun for eruption, will be discussed in Chapter 6.

Irritant Contact Dermatitis
Upon contact irritating substances cause a stinging and burning sensation with some itching. Unlike allergy-producing contact chemicals, irritants do not produce bio-chemical reactions. If they are strong and caustic, such as acids or alkalis, they can produce burns or ulcers upon first contact of the skin. Weaker irritants such as soaps and detergents will take repeated exposure to defat the skin, and make it dry, scaly, red and fissured.

The materials that can produce irritation are legion. I cannot mention all of them, but here are some of the more common ones.

Alkali soaps, detergents, shampoos, bubble bath preparations, antiperspirants, depilatories, permanent wave liquids.

Household cleaners: lye, oven cleaners, toilet bowl cleaners, polishes, bleaches, ammonia.

Fruit and vegetable juices.

Rubbing (isopropyl) alcohol, liniments.

Certain chemicals cause a specific reaction which identifies them as the responsible agent. Industrial cutting oils that are chlorinated produce a type of severe acne on the exposed areas. In machinists, arms and legs and the face are affected with horny, black plugs in hair and oil gland pores, along with firm acne-like bumps. This condition is called chloracne. It responds to treatment slowly.

Petroleum oils may also cause a skin pigmentation, and at times a coin-shaped eczema, in the areas of contact.

Avoidance of the irritant is the first and foremost step in treating contact dermatitis. Topical treatment will vary depending on the type of irritation. Common hand irritations, for example, will respond to emollients and mild steroid creams. This treatment will not benefit chloracne. Instead keratolytic creams (those that dissolve scale) such as salicylic acid creams should be used. An oral antibiotic may have to be taken if the acne nodules are infected.

Everything we do involves our hands. They are, therefore, the most common location for contact dermatitis of both kinds. Interestingly, this dermatitis does not affect the palms or palmar side of the finger – at least not initially. The stratum corneum, the thick, topmost layer of our palms, protects them. Chemicals do not penetrate easily through this layer. Consequently, the tops of the hands and sides of the hands and fingers show changes first. The palmar areas will show changes with severe dermatitis.

Allergic Contact Dermatitis

The problem substance causing irritant dermatitis is easy to find, but the one causing an allergy may challenge the wits and patience of the most dedicated dermatologist. There is a time lapse between contact of an allergy-causing chemical and the outbreak of the allergic rash. In the meantime you will most probably have forgotten which of the many things you touch daily may be the problem. If you have had the rash before and know that you have had contact with the same allergen again, or if you have picked a particular plant known to cause allergy, the answer is clear. Usually, it is not.

How do you and your doctor begin to pinpoint the problem? It is important to decide whether you have an irritant contact dermatitis or an allergic one. That should not be too difficult to determine. An irritant will be irritating to everyone who comes in contact with it, while an allergen will sensitize only those people with the greatest susceptibility for developing allergic reactions.

The skin effect from an irritant will be almost immediate – from stinging, burning to caustic burns. There will be no immediate effect from an allergen (the substance that causes allergy). That takes time to develop. When it does, itching is a prominent symptom.

An irritant contact dermatitis is seldom eczematous. An allergic contact dermatitis is always eczematous, with vesicles that soon combine to form moist patches. Autosensitiz-ation reactions (secondary rashes on uninvolved parts of the body) occur in the latter dermatitis, not in the former. Reactions from an irritant reflect the substance involved:

81

detergents will cause chapping; acids, caustic burns; and cutting oils, acne-type eruptions.

An allergic contact dermatitis may be more visually defined as to origin. A reaction to an elastic band in shorts will cause a rash in the shape of a band around the waist. Configurations like this, in addition to causing interesting patterns, also make the search for the allergen easier. Irritants as a rule will not show specific, well-defined shapes, since they are too irritating and damaging for the patient to tolerate for very long.

How Do You Develop Contact Allergy?

Exposure to the chemical ingredient is necessary. You may use or work with something a few times and develop an allergy, or it may take months and years of exposure before you develop an allergic reaction. A florist may suddenly get an allergy to chrysanthemums, although he or she has been handling them for a long time. In other words, individual susceptibility to an allergen varies. Likewise, the sensitizing potential of a substance varies. Some are potent sensitizers, others are not. Dinitrochlorobenzene (DNCB) is a chemical that sensitizes almost everyone who comes in contact with it, but hydrocortisone rarely sensitizes a person. DNCB is of interest because it is used in medical research to test a patient's ability to be skin sensitized. A weak or negative response in patients with atopic dermatitis gives evidence of the decreased ability to get skin allergies in this condition.

Predisposing factors will enhance your chances of being sensitized. Individual tendency is one of them. Local conditions are another. The production of soggy, macerated skin from frequent exposure to water will permit substances to penetrate more easily. Abraded, scratched skin is also more vulnerable.

Sensitizing substances are small, active chemicals that

penetrate the skin readily. They bind with a skin protein to form a biochemical called an antigen. This antigen is immunologically offensive to the body, which forms an antibody to counteract the antigen. An antigen-antibody reaction occurs through the interaction of several cells. This takes time to develop and is therefore known as a 'delayed hypersensitivity' reaction. A white blood cell, presumably influenced by the thymus gland, and therefore called T lymphocyte, is important to the process.

The antigen-antibody (Ag-Ab) complex finally reaches a stage where it causes a dermatitis at the place of contact. Initial sensitization, or development of reactive Ag-Ab complexes, takes seven to fourteen days. In this interval your skin will look perfectly normal. As discussed, this initial sensitization may not occur until days, months, sometimes years, of exposure to a substance.

Once you have been sensitized, a second exposure to the allergen will trigger the rash much sooner, anywhere from twelve to forty-eight hours. Subsequent exposures will always occur within this time frame, but probably at the shorter end because of your greater sensitivity at this point. It takes a certain amount of time for the biochemical Ag-Ab reaction to take place even in a highly sensitized person.

Areas of Body Involved and Substances Causing Allergies in These Regions

Any part of the body can develop a contact dermatitis, although certain areas are more readily sensitized than others. The skin of the genital and eyelid areas tends to be more reactive.

Contact dermatitis occurs on the hands most frequently, but not because they are more sensitive. They simply are at higher risk, being exposed to all sorts of things. Ninety per cent of occupational contact rashes are on the hands. The hands show allergies, commonly, to the chromates in cement, nickel in electroplating, rubber chemicals found in rubber gloves and to plant substances. There are also many other substances that may cause allergies, but these are less frequent and too numerous to mention.

The head and neck can develop allergies to cosmetics, perfumes, hair dyes and sprays and costume jewellery. Nickel is the chemical in the latter that causes sensitization.

The eyelids can be sensitized by substances transmitted to them by the hands. Plant allergies and allergy to fingernail polish can present this way. Since the hands are more resistant, they may be spared. The eruption, therefore, could be confusing to you and your doctor unless you are aware of this pattern. Cosmetics such as mascara and eyeliner may cause problems. Thiomerasol in soft contact lens soaking solution can also sensitize.

The lips are primarily affected by lipsticks, toothpastes (primarily coloured ones), mouthwashes and limes.

The trunk primarily shows allergies to clothes, perfumes, to nickel in bra clips, zips and suspender clips.

Crease-resistant clothes will contain formaldehyde which is a sensitizer. It is also added to clothes to increase the bulk of inexpensive fabrics. Washing crease-resistant clothes and synthetics before wearing them will get rid of residual formalin and cut down the risk of allergy.

Rubber in elasticized garments is another allergen. The rubbing and chafing from these articles further enhances the potential for sensitivity. Bra straps, elastic bands and girdles fall into this group.

Armpits are susceptible to allergies from deodorants, perfumes and clothes. Heavy sweating produces irritation and maceration of the skin, which contributes to the susceptibility. Interestingly, for reasons that are unclear, the vault of the armpit is seldom involved with the allergic rash. Some dermatologists believe this is because clothes are not in direct contact with it, while they are with the surrounding skin which does break out.

The arms show reactions to dust, sprays, plants, perfumes, nickel in costume jewellery and wrist watches. The chemicals in leather or elastic watch bands can also produce allergies.

Crease-resistant clothes, polyesters and synthetics cause problems on the legs; so do depilatories, plants, cement or plaster dust that has permeated workers' trousers.

The feet will show reactions to the dye or formalin in socks, and react to chemical substances in shoes. Chemicals used in the making of the rubber toe-box, cements and chemicals used in tanning shoe leather are usually offending agents. Heavy sweating is a predisposing factor in shoe allergies. Feet are similar to hands in reactivity. The soles are relatively impervious to penetration by chemical allergens. Therefore, the eruption will appear first on the tops of the toes and the instep. A shoe patch test kit is available for testing to a specific chemical.

The genital and anal area is often affected by allergic reactions. The characteristic warmth and moisture in the region encourage sensitization. Occlusive clothing will further increase the risk. Some sensitizers are formalin-treated clothes, elastic girdles, elastic panties, nylon, perfumes. Medications used in the area may likewise sensitize. Be aware of rectal suppositories containing benzocaine and other anaesthetic 'caine' derivatives. Anti-infective preparations containing neomycin and hydroxyquinoline (Vioform) may also sensitize.

A Summary: Chemicals that Commonly Cause Allergic Dermatitis and Where they are Found

Nickel is a potent sensitizer and most common cause of allergic contact dermatitis. It is combined with cobalt to make costume jewellery and many other metal articles. Hair pins, garter clips, necklaces, watches, scissors, car door handles are a few of the myriad objects that contain this ubiquitous substance. Jewellers, by the nature of their profession, would be at high risk.

Casual contact will not produce sensitivity. Repeated rubbing and abrasion of the skin is needed. Concomitant sensitivity to nickel and cobalt is common, since the two exist together.

Unlike other contact allergens, nickel affects the palms, and therefore is an exception to the rule that most contact dermatitis begins on the sides and tops of the hands.

Chromates. The base substance is chromium. Chromates are the other exception to the rule. They also can sensitize the palms and soles first. They are commonly found in cement, paint, matches, leather (hat bands, sandals), varnishes, fur dyes. Masons and tanners are at high risk.

Rubber. Natural rubber itself does not sensitize, but synthetic rubber does. However, the elastic in clothing contains a combination of synthetic and natural rubber. The culprits are chemical accelerators and antioxidants used in the manufacture of rubber compounds. The accelerators increase the vulcanization of rubber. The antioxidants are preservatives. (Vulcanization, in case you do not know, is a process by which rubber is treated to increase its strength and elasticity.)

It has been discovered that laundry bleach in the wash will change the rubber in elastic-containing garments into a very potent sensitizer. When you wash your girdles, panties, bra, etcetera, avoid bleach.

Plants. In Great Britain, primrose is the most common plant source of allergic contact dermatitis. The responsible substance is an oleoresin, called Primulin, which is present in the glandular hairs of the plant. The rash will occur on the fingers and is often transmitted to the neck and face.

Philodendron, English ivy and tulips are a few others that will cause contact eczema. On the Scilly Isles, flower-handlers have developed a dermatitis to daffodils and narcissi.

Rhus dermatitis, caused by poison ivy and poison oak, is the most common plant rash in the United States.

Organic dye. Paraphenylenediamine (PPD) is a substance found commonly around us, and is a strong sensitizer. Permanent hair dyes, dyed furs, leather (shoes, wrist bands) all contain it. PPD exhibits *cross reactivity*. It is important to remember this. Once sensitized by it, you can also be sensitized to substances that contain similar chemical structures. Anaesthetics such as procaine and benzocaine and sulphonamide medications cross-react with PPD.

Formalin or formaldehyde. As already mentioned this is common in crease-resistant fabrics. When you enter a store, you can sometimes detect its acrid smell. It is a common cause of problems in the textile industry. It is also found in polishes and glues, and is used as a preservative in cosmetics.

Plastics and glues. These most often cause occupational problems in aeroplane workers, cabinet makers, artists and painters. The problem agents are epoxy resins, usually creating trouble prior to mixing with a hardener. Acrylates are being used in industry and can cause dermatitis. Printers are at risk.

Cosmetics. The dyes and perfumes in lipsticks, the preservatives in eye make-up can sensitize. Nail lacquers which have sulphonamides and formalin, plus resins, sensitize fairly often. Artificial nails and nail hardeners also cause reactions and can cause secondary infection and destruction of the nails. But considering the widespread use of cosmetics, the percentage of allergic reactions is small.

Medications. I have already mentioned the most common sensitizers: neomycin, topical antihistamines, anaesthetics, Vioform (hydroxyquinoline). Preservatives such as parabens and formalin are used in cream preparations and can sensitize. Many of the steroid ointments contain parabens, but this is a rare cause of sensitization. Lanolin, which has been mentioned as a sensitizer, rarely sensitizes normal skin. The skin has to be broken or eczematous.

Identifying the Allergen

Many times one has to be a Sherlock Holmes to figure out which of the many substances could be the problem. The doctor may ask you to keep a diary of everything with which you come in contact. That is tedious, but it might provide important information.

The best and easiest way to find out what may be causing your dermatitis is for the doctor to do a patch test.

Patch testing. The testing should never be done while there is an active rash, since a positive reaction will probably make the dermatitis worse. Even after the rash has cleared, the skin will be extra-sensitive for a while and should be allowed to recover fully. Also, the test should not be done on the same skin where there was a recent allergic rash.

The preferred site for the patch tests is the middle of the back.

A simple, somewhat crude method of testing would be for the doctor to take a dilute, not irritating, solution made from the substance in question, and apply it to a square centimetre of lint. This would then be applied to normal skin, covered with cellophane and taped in place with one of the micropore hypoallergenic surgical tapes (Dermicel), or with Sellotape.

The testing is usually not done this way, as most skin doctors and clinics have a special skin allergy testing kit, which contains the most common allergens in appropriate concentrations. These can be applied on an aluminium-foil-backed square and taped in place. Some places use a Finn chamber which is a small circular flat metal container on a hypoallergenic tape backing. The allergen is placed in the chamber and taped in place. One or several of these can be taped at once. Thus, several allergens can be tested simultaneously (see Fig. 8).

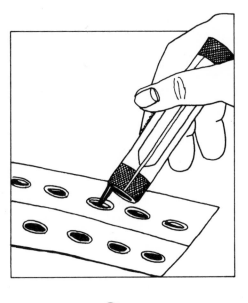

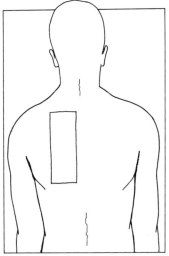

Fig. 8   Patch Testing: Finn Chamber Method
A   Individual allergens to be tested are placed in the small Finn
      chambers which come mounted on a Scanpore tape strip.
B   The prepared Scanpore tape is applied on to the back for patch
      testing. The back is a typical test site. After 48-72 hours the test is
      read. A positive allergic reaction will be characterized by several
      small, itchy blisters on a red base.

The patch tests should be kept in place for forty-eight hours and read at this time. They should be removed earlier only if there is an intense reaction before the forty-eight hours are up. If there is no reaction or a minimal reaction, the patch should be kept in place for another twenty-four hours and then read again. A positive test is one in which there is redness, swelling and tiny 'sago-grain' blisters, accompanied by itching; in other words, a typical early acute dermatitis, which developed in reaction to the allergen.

Unfortunately, patch testing is not 100 per cent accurate, because the identical conditions that caused the original allergic rash cannot be duplicated on the back with the test allergen. However, the test is positive in a majority of patients tested, and is a helpful tool in finding the cause of an allergic dermatitis.

Skin-testing kits. The group of chemicals in the kit are a result of intensive research by the International Contact Dermatitis Research Group. These substances, with the most likely sources, are as follows:

ALLERGEN	CONTACT SOURCE
Potassium dichromate 0.5%	Cement, anti-rust agents, plating dyes, bleaches, photographic chemicals, laboratory chemicals
Cobalt chloride 1%	Dyes, cement, clay, anti-corrosives, animal feeds
Nickel sulphate 5%	Cheap jewellery, metals, plating

Formaldehyde (in water) 2%	Preservatives, cosmetics, shampoos, adhesives, leather tanning, photography, laboratory fixative, anti-fungus, disinfectant, anti-perspirant (powders, solutions), inner soles
Paraphenylenediamine 1%	Anti-oxidants, photographic chemicals, cosmetic dyes
Balsam of Peru 25%	Perfumes, medicaments
Neomycin sulphate 20%	Anti-infective ointments
Parabens (methyl-, ethyl-, propyl-, butyl-, benzyl-, 3% each) 15% total	Preservatives in medicaments or cosmetics, food preservatives
Chinoform 5%	Medicaments
Colophony 20%	Adhesives in strapping, polishes, printing ink, violin rosin, filling material, soap, rubber and plastics
Wood tars (pine, beech, juniper, birch, 3% each) 12% total	Woods, medicaments
Wool alcohols 30%	Lanolin, medicaments, cosmetics
Epoxy resin 1%	Adhesives, flooring, anti-rust paint
Mercapto-mix (mixture of four chemicals, 0.5% each) 2% total	Rubber accelerators, oils

Thiuram-mix (mixture of four chemicals, 0.25%) 1% total	Biocides – fruit, nuts, mushrooms, rose sprays – rubber accelerator
PPD-mix (mixture of three chemicals, 0.10%, 0.25%, 0.25%) 0.6% total	Anti-oxidant, rubber, oils
Naphthyl-mix (mixture of two chemicals, 0.5% each) 1% total	Rubber
Carbo-mix (mixture of three chemicals, 1% each) 3% total	Rubber accelerator
Ethylene diamine dihydrochloride 1%	Medicaments
Fragrance-mix (mixture of eight chemicals, 2% each) 16% total	Perfumes

When the chemical causing your dermatitis is discovered, find out what other substances contain it. You will need to avoid all materials with that sensitizing ingredient in them.

Treatment

Avoidance is the best treatment. Stay away from substances that have given you an allergic rash in the past. If you do contact one of them, wash it off as quickly as possible. This will eliminate the substance available for penetration and will diminish the intensity of the reaction.

You can try barrier hand creams, but they are not very effective. The best barrier is protective clothing. If you have to work with a sensitizer, wear appropriate overalls or gloves. (For instructions regarding the wearing of protective gloves, see p. 65.) Industrial places should have a clean work environment with no problem chemicals lying around or blowing about.

Acute contact dermatitis of moderate to severe intensity is an indication for systemic steroids, either by injection or a short course of oral medicines. This should be curative, because a specific problem, known to be responsive to steroids, is being treated.

Wet compresses with aluminium acetate solution should be used topically. Secondary infections should be treated with systemic antibiotics. An antihistamine may be needed for itching.

For a mild dermatitis, steroids of moderate potency can be used.

Most types of contact dermatitis are acute in nature. If a patient does not get proper treatment or repeated exposures continue, a chronic dermatitis can develop. Treatment is elimination of the contact and administration of steroids, systemic and topical or both. Infection may be a problem and should be treated with antibiotics.

Chapter Four

URTICARIA

Urticaria is the medical name for 'nettle rash', as it is commonly known in Britain; hives is another name for it. Nettle, on contact with the skin causes the typical wheal and flare reaction of urticaria, thus the rash became known as nettle rash. However, many other things can cause the eruption. Therefore, I prefer to use the interchangeable words 'hives' and 'urticaria' in the discussion, since they are less confusing as to origin.

Hives may be either acute or chronic; the causes are similar. An allergic reaction to internal drugs is the most common genesis of urticaria. Streptococcal sore throat, herpes infections and underlying disease, e.g. diabetes, lymphoma, can also produce the condition. The latter is usually of the chronic type. The list of possible causes is long.

The acute state, often, occurs as a sudden eruption to an evident cause, such as oral medication (penicillin), or severe stress in susceptible people, e.g. getting fired. Acute hives commonly disappear after a few days of treatment. However, if the inciting factor persists, so will your hives.

Chronic urticaria may last days, weeks, even months. It may be episodic, disappearing then reappearing at intervals which vary from days to months. Sometimes a year or more elapses between attacks. Usually, you do not recall any obvious causative factor.

Stress-induced hives are more likely to occur in people who have the atopic condition (dermatitis, hay fever, asthma), or who have a family history of it. However, the field of medicine is nothing, if not variable. Stress-related hives can beleaguer a person without a predisposing personal or familial atopic history. In general, urticaria from any source, psychogenic or not, will be made worse by emotional stress.

But before your doctor decides on the diagnosis of nervous strain, he or she should rule out any physical reason for your problem. A thorough clinical history and physical examination should be done. If the urticaria continues over the years, periodic evaluation of your physical health is in order.

Urticaria is characterized by very itchy whitish wheals with surrounding redness (flare). Stinging and burning may be accompanying symptoms. The breaking out occurs anywhere on the body, sometimes in clusters. Frequently, covered areas are affected first, i.e. trunk and thighs. Shortly after the appearance of one group, another will appear somewhere else, while the first group disappears. A hive does not stay in one place for very long. One to eight hours are typical durations. This coming and going is very characteristic.

Their size varies too: 1 to 3 cm is the average, but smaller and larger wheals occur also.

Histamine is the basic substance responsible for urticaria. The mast cell is responsible for histamine; it is pregnant with histamine-containing granules and exists around small cutaneous blood vessels. When certain factors impact on the mast cell, they stimulate its histamine release, thereby creating the wheal and flare reaction.

The raised, whitish quality of the wheal is secondary to fluid which has leaked through capillary walls made permeable by histamine. Small blood vessels in the region become dilated too. This accounts for the erythema, or redness, of the skin around the wheal.

As in most circumstances, nothing is simple. Other implicated biochemical substances in urticaria are heparin, serotonin and kinins. These are breakdown products – polypeptides – of proteins. They act as inflammatory agents, contributing to swelling and pain. Bradykinin is the best-known of them. But histamine is the most important stimulator.

In urticaria, the entire skin becomes sensitized and has the potential of developing the eruption. Pressure, stroking or heat will elicit hives. For example, stroking the skin firmly with a finger or blunt end of a pen will bring out a linear wheal with surrounding red flare along the stroke line. This response is called dermographism or skin writing. In this manner, one can actually 'write' a word on a spacious part of the body, such as the back. In appearance, the skin writing resembles the fluffy letters of sky writing. It is a simple test used by doctors to determine the skin's reactive state.

Treatment

In non-psychogenic urticaria, the physical cause needs to be eliminated: stop the allergy-producing drug, treat the streptococcal sore throat, avoid the offending agent (animal danders, pollens, etcetera), find the underlying disease and so on. At the same time, treatment for urticaria begins.

An injection of 1:1000 epinephrine quickly counteracts the histamine effects of a severe, acute attack of hives. This can be followed by oral antihistamines, and/or a short course of steroids. Antihistamines are the drug of choice when the condition is not too severe.

Antihistamines are, usually, adequate for psychogenic urticaria. In refractory cases, a short course of steroids will be helpful. Tranquillizers may help, too. But these are temporary measures and do not get at the root of the problem. An attempt should be made to deal with the emotional stress in your life, or the wheals will continue.

There may be repressed feelings which you yourself don't recognize. Talking with a sympathetic person, a friend or clinician, may lead you to a recognition of these emotions. The release of tension that follows this recognition is sometimes enough to eliminate hives. Dermatologists report such instances in the office, after they have given a patient time to talk and get to the bottom of the problem (see Chapter 9).

Sweat Urticaria

Sweat urticaria is inherited as a genetic trait. Although it is uncommon, it provides a wonderfully clear-cut example of the effects of nervous stress on the skin. Anything else that induces sweating will also induce hives in this condition, but emotional tension is the most common factor. The hives occur in a most specific pattern, which I will describe shortly.

Elucidation of the physiological mechanism by which sweat causes hives is a credit to medical investigation. When a person is subject to emotional stress, nervous impulses go out from the brain, eventually to reach the nerve endings in the skin. These endings are the parasympathetic part of the autonomic nervous system, which controls sweating through the release of a hormonal substance, acetylcholine. The latter then stimulates the release of sweat. In medical circles, sweat urticaria is, therefore, also called 'cholinergic' urticaria.

Sweat causes the release of hives but, paradoxically, around fine body hair rather than around the sweat glands, which would seem the logical place for the reaction. Why is this so?

The answer is a toxic compound formed by the reaction of sweat and sebum, the greasy substance of the skin's oil glands. Sweat acts indirectly through this compound. Since the oil gland empties into the hair opening or pore, the toxic substance finds its way to the base of the hair. Here, it acts on the mast cells and *voilà!* – hives erupt on the skin surface around the hair.

The hives are tiny, 1 to 3 mm, and discrete. This, plus their location, is a contrast to common urticaria. The wheals are extremely itchy, last for about thirty to ninety minutes, and are followed by a refractory period of twenty-four hours.

When the refractory period is over, the skin becomes reactive again. The skin stroke test will demonstrate this nicely, by the production of the characteristic wheal with a large flare.

Although antihistamines in adequate doses will control the problem, the better drug, and drug of choice, is hydroxyzine. It controls effectively, but does not cure. That depends on relief from psychogenic problems.

Chapter Five

ITCH

Itching (the Latin name is *pruritus*) is the most important and prevalent symptom in dermatitis. It is exclusive to the skin. No other organs are so affected. It can appear without any noticeable skin changes, either as a generalized or localized itch. Ear canals, eyelids, nostrils, anal and genital areas, the 'itch spots' of the body, are more susceptible than other parts.

Individual reactions to itching stimuli vary. Some people will itch a lot, others not very much. Patterns of itching, also, vary from person to person. Itching, without a preceding rash, may localize in one area, e.g. the ear canal in one person, and the anal area in another.

Itching may be continuous or episodic. It may occur in bursts, driving a person into a fit of scratching. Itching, severe enough to wake a person at night, is more likely to be due to an underlying disease, rather than to psychogenic orgin.

I can be consistent in stating that there are many variations and variables to the sensation of itching, which is why it is so difficult to quantify, both as a clinical and physiological process. Attempts have been and are being made, but it is too complex, variable and subject to too many ambiguous individual interpretations to be satisfactory for laboratory study.

We know it is mediated through neural and biochemical interactions, travelling along the same nerve fibres that transmit touch, hot and cold sensations. In the brain, a sensory impulse will be transmitted to a motor impulse that causes the physical act of scratching. Biochemical substances – histamine, kinins, proteases among them – play a role in the skin. For our purposes, we need to know that itching is a subjective sensation, controlled and affected by a complex of psychological, neural and biochemical factors.

Causes of Generalized Itch

Many things cause itching or contribute to it. I can discuss only the more important and frequent ones. Bear in mind that more than one of the things under discussion may, concurrently, contribute to itching.

Skin diseases. All of the dermatitis group produce itch. Urticaria is often a further extension of the itching problem. Common infestations of the skin – lice and scabies – cause itch.

Certain uncommon skin diseases produce severe itching. One of them, *dermatitis herpetiformis,* is characterized by discrete small red papules and blisters that erupt typically between the shoulders, on the buttocks and other typical regions. These can drive the patient 'crazy' with itch. Fortunately, the cause, a biochemical defect, has been discovered. Specific medicine exists to clear and control the problem (see p. 143).

Lichen planus is another uncommon skin disease that produces severe itching. Small, purplish polygonal-shaped papules erupt on the trunk and limbs. The surfaces of the lesions are smooth and shiny. Unlike the eczemas, there are no moist lesions. The cause is unknown, and the treatment is not terribly effective. Steroids are prescribed with mixed results. The eruption usually runs its course of several months to years and spontaneously resolves. The break-out is sometimes stress-induced. Women of thirty or older are more likely to develop this rash.

Climatic conditions. Environments of low humidity dry

the skin and create a condition for itching. Central heating, dry, cold weather, a dry desert environment, hot dry winds and wind chill factors in cold climates will all dry the skin.

Inefficient sweating. Certain individuals, notably those with atopic tendencies, but not invariably, will be unable to sweat normally in high humidity. This inability to cool the skin physiologically will cause itching.

Heat. Overheating the body through excessive physical exertion will aggravate itch. So will hot baths, saunas and heating pads or electric blankets. The rule is to stay cool.

Substances on the skin. All the contact irritants and allergens fall into this group. Fine fibreglass particles can cause severe itch. Certain danders and dusts will also. Of the latter, sawdust, plaster and cement dust can be factors. Rubbing (isopropyl) alcohol, preparations containing tincture of isopropyl alcohol, will dry the skin and make it itch. Soaps and detergents are itch-inducing irritants.

Clothing. Occlusive, heavy clothing will increase heat and rubbing of the skin and aggravate itch. Woollens, nylons, polyesters may cause itch. Cotton does not, unless it has been treated to be crease-resistant. Clothing laundered with too much detergent may cause itch.

Ageing. As we get older, the skin gets drier and thinner. Both of these changes make the skin more vulnerable to irritants and itching.

Internal disease. Overactive and underactive thyroid problems, renal disease, the jaundice of liver disease, diabetes, internal cancers and lymphomas can be associated with itching. Sometimes, intractable itching is the first sign of internal disease. Lymphomas may present this way.

Stimulants. Coffee, tea, chocolate, tobacco, alcohol and drugs may all cause itch. Hyper-excitement and lack of sleep can too.

Psychological. Emotional instability, tension, anxiety, frustration, fear, anger, resentment, shame – any emotional reaction can be displaced to the skin with resultant generalized or local itching.

Medicines. Diazides, used in hypertension treatment, are an example of medicines which can produce itch.

Common Itch Factors in Localized Body Regions

Before going on to a discussion of psychosomatic itching, I want to summarize the most prevalent causes of itching in specific body areas. Nervous stress can cause or worsen itching in all these parts.

In the *scalp*, eczemas, seborrhoeic dermatitis (advanced dandruff) and lice are common itch-inducing problems. Psoriasis, which often afflicts the scalp, does not itch. However, everyone has a different tolerance for itch, or different itch threshold. Those with a low itch threshold (often anxious, frustrated people), will have an itching problem with psoriasis, regardless of its location. For them, scalp involvement can be very pruritic.

The *ears*, primarily the ear canals, itch from eczemas, severe dandruff problems and psoriasis.

Common causes of itchy *eyelids* are eczemas, seborrhoeic dermatitis, contact irritants, allergens (dust and danders), plus nervous stress.

Hay fever most often creates itching of the *nose* and eyes. Dry skin will make nostrils itch. Sjogren's syndrome, a condition which can develop in long-standing rheumatoid arthritis, shows diminished sweating and will make nostrils itch.

The *upper chest* over the breastbone is a common site for seborrhoeic dermatitis (see pp. 123–8). This plus eczemas can create itching here.

The *nipples* react with itch to noxious contactants, eczemas and psychosomatic itching.

Forearms: irritants, allergens, dermatitis, hives and scabies are common itch-producing problems.

Many things cause itching of the *hands*. Contact dermatitis (see pp. 79 ff) and other eczemas are the most common. Psoriasis affects the hands and may itch in certain people. Scabies, occurring in the finger webs and around the wrists, can provoke severe itching.

Varicose vein dermatitis, atopic dermatitis, nummular dermatitis, asteatotic dermatitis and dry skin commonly cause itching of the *legs*.

The *anal and genital area* in general is more likely to develop itch and skin sensitivity than other parts of the body. There are many possible etiological sources. Underlying metabolic diseases, e.g. diabetes, also vaginal infections and topical medications may produce itch. Certain internal medicines may cause pruritus. In this group, the tetracyclines are often implicated. They predispose the patient to yeast infection, which may contribute to the itch. The dermatitis and contact dermatitis group, of course, cause itching in this region.

Certain infestations – in particular, lice and threadworms – must be considered. The nits and lice are seen in the pubic and upper inner thigh hair. The excrement of the lice, visible as black specks, is irritating to the skin and causes itching. Recognition should be easy. Treatment with Kwell lotion is curative.

Threadworms may be missed if the doctor does not think of them. Although anyone can get them, they are most common in children. Sellotape pressed around the anal area will pick up the eggs of the threadworms. When the tape is put on a glass slide and examined microscopically, the eggs will be evident. Once diagnosis is made, specific treatment eliminates threadworms and cures the itch.

The anal and genital area may be affected by itching of a psychogenic nature. However, a thorough physical examination should always be done first to rule out any other causes.

Psychosomatic Itching

A continuous, chronic itch without evident cause may be psychological in origin. However, the diagnosis can be an excuse for ignorance on the part of the doctor. It is easy to say the itch is 'just nerves', if the doctor can not find anything else or is too busy to look into the problem carefully.

Even if it is 'just nerves', itching should not be dismissed lightly. It can be a disruptive and frustrating symptom – driving sufferers to distraction.

Before diagnosing psychogenic itch, your doctor should ask certain questions: 'Describe the itching. Where is it? When does it occur – day or night?' Itching waking you from sleep probably has an underlying physical cause. 'Is it seasonal?' An itch in winter is often due to dry skin. 'Do mental or physical activities make it worse? Is there a relationship between the itch and something else?' Certain emotions or activities may aggravate it.

The physical examination should include a complete blood count with examination for abnormal cells. A sedimentation rate, urine and stool examination and a chest X-ray should all be done. These are routine. Additionally, blood tests to examine the liver, kidney and thyroid should be done. If indicated, your doctor may want to do certain special studies – blood to test your immune system or more sophisticated thyroid tests. A serum iron test may be advisable. Sometimes, a decreased level of iron in the serum will cause itching when the haemoglobin level is normal. Your examination will undoubtedly be fine, and you will be pronounced healthy. The comfort of that knowledge should, in itself, make you feel better.

Psychosomatic itching has certain characteristics. There is no overt cause. It is widespread, or localized to a symbolically significant area – the nipples, scrotum, vulva, eyelids.

The intensity of itching is connected with the emotions of the individual. Conflict, anger, resentment will aggravate the itch. Repeated rubbing and scratching may cause thickening of the skin with production of localized eczema.

A patient's description of the itch may be exaggerated and bizarre, not coinciding with any physiological pattern. 'It spreads from my forehead, down to my neck'; 'I thought I was going to choke – electricity was passing through my body. It went out my big toes. I didn't have any more itch until the next morning.'

Many times, evidence of scratching is slight, and does not coincide with the described severity of the itch. On the other hand, there may be marked scratch and gouge marks.

Psychogenic itch rarely disturbs sleep unless it is in the genital and anal area. Then intense gouging and scratching can occur, drawing blood. The patient may not be aware of this activity until morning, when blood stains are visible on pyjamas.

All itch, whether psychogenic or not, is worse at night, just before falling asleep. This is definitely noticeable in scabies.

Several reasons are postulated for the nocturnal increase in itching: there are fewer distractions at night, therefore one is more aware of itching; the section of the nervous system that controls itching (parasympathetic system) is more active. Also, the skin blood vessels dilate at the end of the day, giving off more heat. Metabolism is also higher after a day's activity. The increased body heat from these sources, plus increase in heat from bed covers, all add to the itch.

Eroticism is an element of itching. Rubbing and scratching provide the patient with pleasurable sensations, even when carried to the point of skin damage. The pain goes unnoticed until after the itch stops. Paroxysmal bouts of itching, that afflict the sufferer, are likened to orgasms of the skin. European dermatologists call it *orgasme cutané*.

Treatment
Sedatives, tranquillizers and antihistamines are more effec-

tive in control than topical medications. But even this systemic treatment does not resolve the itch, and there is always the danger of addiction to repeated use of sedatives or tranquillizers.

At best, psychosomatic itch is not easy to manage. Insight alone does not provide a cure, although it is an important step in that direction. The itch continues until the emotional problem causing it goes away, or you learn to deal with repressed feelings. Psychotherapy is, usually, the best approach. There are reports of patients, under the guidance of sympathetic doctors, recalling repressed emotions with the resultant cessation of itching.

Chapter Six

RELATED
AND RELEVANT
CONDITIONS

Now I want to discuss several skin diseases which either have dermatitis as one of their components, or are totally different entities that may sometimes be confused with the dermatitis group.

PHOTODERMATITIS

Sunlight acting upon substances on or in the skin can produce an allergic dermatitis which is mediated through the body's immune system; or it can produce a phototoxic eruption. The latter has the characteristics of a severe sunburn and is *not* mediated by the immune system.

Photoallergic Contact Dermatitis
This presents as a typical acute or subacute dermatitis on a sun-exposed area of the body. Antibacterial compounds (primarily halogenated sulphur chemicals) present in antibacterial soaps, perfumes, cosmetics, cleaning agents and topical medications are the main culprits interacting with sunlight to produce photoallergic contact dermatitis.

The wavelength of light responsible for sensitivity is called the 'Action Spectrum'. This action spectrum is in the long ultraviolet light to visible light range. For a reaction to take place, the spectrum has to encompass the absorption range of the photosensitizing chemical. Each chemical has its own specific absorption range.

Once the sunlight reacts with this photosensitizer, the immunological process is the same as for regular allergic contact dermatitis (see pp. 79 ff.). A delayed hypersensitivity reaction occurs, during which your body is primed by the formation of antibodies to the photosensitizer. When a subsequent sensitizing exposure occurs, the skin will erupt within twenty-four to forty-eight hours with an acute dermatitis involving the sun-exposed area. The presence of a small amount of photosensitizer is all that is required for this latter reaction. Itching and burning are associated symptoms.

Some people become persistent light reactors following their initial bout of photodermatitis. Even after the photosensitizers are gone, they continue to have symptoms of itching and/or recurrent bouts of dermatitis in the sun-exposed areas. This may go on for months, even years. Sulphur substances (halogenated salicylanilides, found in deodorant soaps and other deodorant preparations) most often set the patient up for this type of problem.

An interesting localized photoallergy occurs in tattoos containing the yellow sulphide substance, cadmium sulphide. Other colours in the tattoo pigment do not provoke a reaction to sunlight.

Treatment for photoallergic contact dermatitis is the same as for other eczemas: astringent compresses to dry the acute moist dermatitis and bland corticosteroid creams or ointments. In addition, you have to avoid the sun as much as possible, especially during its peak intensity of 10 a.m. to 2 p.m. In particular, this is critical when the dermatitis is acute. Naturally, avoid the photoallergy-causing substance.

When you go out, sunscreens should be applied. The most effective ones contain PABA (para-aminobenzoic acid) and have a sun-protective factor of 15 or greater. Bear in mind that PABA takes two hours to become effective after application. However, it also has the advantage of building stores in the epidermis. Therefore, repeated applications will provide better protection. If the dermatitis is moist, you will probably not be able to apply sunscreens comfortably: they may be too messy or cause stinging of the open areas. In this case, it is best to avoid the sun. Wear protective clothing if you need to go out. Begin sunscreen applications when the rash has cleared.

Once the dermatitis has gone and the skin is no longer reactive, patch testing can be done to pinpoint the sensitizer. First, a regular patch test is applied and read in forty-eight hours to determine if the substance, by itself, is an allergen. If it is not, the site is then exposed to the 'action spectrum' wavelength of UV light necessary to activate the chemical. The site is read again in another forty-eight hours.

Photoallergy from Internal Sources

Photoallergic reactions from internal drugs, e.g. sulphur, do not always present as dermatitis reactions. Instead, they may appear as individual blisters and be accompanied with fever and other systemic symptoms. Also these reactions may not stay confined to the sun-exposed areas. They begin here, but through the process of autosensitization (see pp. 29 ff.) can spread to other parts of the body. Autosensitization can also occur in photoallergic contact dermatitis, through the same mechanisms as discussed in atopic dermatitis.

There also exist uncommon genetically-determined internal diseases that produce abnormal biochemicals which sensitize the skin against the sun. Most of these chemicals are 'porphyrins', which normally function in red blood cell formation. However, the normal biochemical process goes awry and certain kinds of porphyrins spill into the blood, urine and skin. The affected skin blisters on sun exposure, or may develop eczema-type eruptions, which over a period of time leave thickening of the involved skin and scarring.

Phototoxic Dermatitis

In contrast to photoallergic contact dermatitis, a phototoxic reaction is caused by a substance that enhances the sunburn effect of sunlight, but does not cause a dermatitis. Since the immune system is not affected, there is no substantial delay in response. A sunburn of varying intensity can occur, depending on the potency of the toxin and its quantity on the skin. The response can be a mild redness to extreme redness with blister formation. The acute reaction leaves behind a residual pigmentation which can take several weeks to clear.

The toxic sunburn occurs two to six hours after initial exposure. Like most sunburns, it reaches its peak at about twenty-four hours.

Coal tar is a common toxic photosensitizer – causing a burn and leaving hyperpigmentation behind. Its phototoxic activity has been turned to advantage in the treatment of psoriasis. When applied to psoriatic plaques, it hastens ultraviolet light action and resolution of the psoriasis.

Many plants contain phototoxic substances called psoralens. The crushed leaves and stems of these plants will release the compound. Once on the skin, psoralen causes the typical toxic sunburn reaction at the exposure site. Psoralen chemicals have been refined for use in the oral treatment of psoriasis, as tablets which enhance the action of ultraviolet light on psoriatic lesions.

The following plants may cause phototoxic reactions: giant hogweed, fig, cowslip, parsley, fennel, dill, wild parsnip, garden carrot, angelica, buttercup, lime bergamot, lime, St John's wort, and pink celery rot. The effect of the latter is due to a psoralen containing fungus which causes the celery rot.

Certain colognes and perfumes, e.g. Shalimar, contain

bergaptens or oil of bergamot which is a source of psoralens. When applied to the skin and exposed to sun, a typical sunburn occurs at the site of application.

Frequent photosensitizers are sulphur compounds, containing a sulphide radical. They may cause both toxic and allergic reactions, either upon local application to the skin or when taken internally. You should be aware of this when taking oral sulphur medication for infections or other ailments. Because they are highly sensitizing, topical sulphur medications are no longer formulated. However, oral sulphur medicines are in common use. Not only are they a source of photoallergy but of allergic reactions in general.

COMMON PHOTOSENSITIZERS

Inducers of Phototoxicity

Oral	Topical
Antibiotics	Coal Tar Derivatives
Demeclocycline	Acridine
(Declomycin)	Anthracene
Tetracycline (rarely)	Phenanthrene
Sulfonamides	Pyridine
Nalidixic acid (NegGram)	Crude coal tar
Griseofulvin (infrequently)	Furocoumarins (psoralens)
Furocoumarins (psoralens)	Methoxsalen (8-MOP) in
Methoxsalen (Oxsoralen)	lime, rue, orange, celery,
Trimethylpsoralen	dill, anise, or mokihana
(Trisoralen)	berry.
Dyes	Bergapten
Acridine	(5-methoxypsoralen) in
Eosin	oil of bergamot
Calcium cyclamate	

Inducers of Photoallergy

Oral ('Photodrug')	Topical ('Photocontact')
Diuretics	Antimicrobials
Chlorothiazides (Diuril,	Bithionol
Hydrodiuril)	Sulfathiazole
Quinethazine (Hydromox)	Halogenated salicylanilides
	and carbanilides
Antidiabetics (Drugs used in	Hexachlorophene (usually
treating Diabetes mellitus)	only secondary sensitizer)
Chlorpropamide (Diabinese)	
Tolbutamide (Orinase)	Antihistamines
	Diphenhydramine?
Phenothiazines (Tranquillizers	(Benadryl)
and anti-vomit medicines)	
Chlorpromazine	
(Thorazine)	
Promazine (Sparine)	
Perchlorperazine	
(Compazine)	
Promethazine (Phenergan)	
Trifluoperazine (Stelazine)	

PITYRIASIS ALBA (WHITE SCALING)

This common and relatively innocuous problem is believed by many dermatologists to be a manifestation of atopic dermatitis. This assumption is based on observation. Children or young adults with dry skin or atopic tendencies often develop superficial dry, whitish scaling patches on their cheeks and sides of their arms. Early dermatologists gave the Latin name *pityriasis alba* to this condition.

If you have it, be reassured it is not serious. Treatment is uncomplicated. Bland skin creams (see List 1, pages 45–7) applied two or three times daily may be sufficient treatment. If not, a mild salicylic acid cream should be effective. When a doctor chooses steroid treatment, a one per cent hydrocortisone cream or ointment is adequate.

PITYRIASIS ROSEA (ROSY SCALING)

Pityriasis rosea is a relatively common eruption, occurring principally in the spring and autumn months. Usually, it affects young people between the ages of fifteen to forty. Because it presents as oval, pink scaling patches, it is sometimes mistaken for discoid dermatitis, ringworm or seborrhoeic dermatitis, which I will discuss later.

However, to a knowledgeable person, *pityriasis rosea*, or PR as it is known among initiates, is a distinctive entity which should be easy to diagnose.

A 'herald' patch, about 2 cm or so across appears, preferentially on the trunk or thighs. It is a pink to salmon-coloured oval with a fine scale that tends to clear in the middle as the lesion ages and forms a fringed peripheral edge or collarette. At this point, the herald patch may be mistaken for a lesion of early discoid dermatitis or ringworm. Unlike the former, however, it does not itch, nor show a moist dermatitis. Ringworm may be hard to differentiate without microscopically examining a scraping that reveals the fungal elements.

A week or two after the herald patch appears, an eruption of smaller but similar lesions, 1 to 2 cm in diameter, will appear, most heavily on the trunk, then on the extremities. Typically, these have a diagonal, 'Christmas-tree' distribution on the back. This identifying appearance along with the herald patch will tell you the diagnosis.

Occasionally, the eruption occurs without evidence of a herald patch. It may be vesicular and then, indeed, resembles discoid dermatitis. But the latter occurs in older patients and itches. The former, vesicular PR, is more common in children than adults, and usually does not itch. However, there are always those patients who disprove the rule.

The distribution of seborrhoeic dermatitis is different from PR, and the lesions are not as discrete and well demarcated. PR does not affect the scalp, while seborrhoeic dermatitis produces scaling. Actually, if one understands the difference between these two skin diseases, there is no reason to confuse them.

The origin of PR is a mystery. The current hypothesis implicates an infection, possibly a virus, as the etiologic agent. The disease is self-limited, usually resolving on its own within eight weeks. Sunlight clears it sooner. If there is itch, Aveenol oatmeal baths can be taken. Hydrocortisone cream can assist the involution and relieve minor itching.

RINGWORM INFECTIONS

This infection has absolutely nothing to do with worms. It is a superficial fungus infection caused by a variety of fungal organisms which can infect any hair-bearing part of the body. The scalp can be involved, as well as the rest of the body, which is covered with fine (lanugo) hair.

Ringworm of the Body (*Tinea corporis*)
Infected dogs or cats are a common infectious source for humans. But you can also pick up the disease through close contact with someone who harbours the organism. Children easily catch it from each other through play and by sharing items of clothing. Early lesions often begin on the arms and legs, but can occur anywhere.

The infection begins as a pink or pinkish tan circle or ring. Actually, most of the lesions are more oval than round. They have a border, consisting of tiny vesicles. The middle of the lesion shows scaling. As the lesions spread outwards, the vesicular border provides the leading edge. I suppose this outward travel through the skin within the shape of a circle is why the name 'ringworm' was coined by the non-medical person.

As the lesion expands it clears in the centre. However, some scaling persists and may extend to the border. In the acute stage there may be itching and a resemblance to discoid dermatitis.

A skin scraping and fungus culture make the diagnosis. With a blade, the doctor or laboratory technician scrapes off the peripheral vesicles with their scales and places them on a glass slide with a drop or two of 10 per cent potassium hydroxide. A glass cover slip is then applied, the preparation is passed through a flame a couple of times and examined under a microscope. Hyphal elements are usually visible. To identify the organism specifically, a similar scraping should be done and placed in a culture medium. Growth will occur in two to three weeks. However, the doctor can begin treatment as soon as he or she makes the diagnosis clinically or microscopically. The result of the culture is, basically, a confirmation of the diagnosis, and is helpful in identifying an unusual or resistant strain of fungus.

Treatment. For limited lesions, topical antifungal treatment should be adequate. Clotrimazole and miconazole are preparations of choice. If the lesions prove resistant, oral griseofulvin can be prescribed.

Ringworm of the Scalp (*Tinea capitis*)
The same organisms which cause skin infections may also involve the scalp. Children are, primarily, affected; adults seldom. The infection is passed from child to child through sharing of combs, hairbrushes or caps.

Scaly patches with vesicles occur on the scalp and scaly papules arise around hairs. Sometimes a sensitivity reaction occurs in the scalp as a response to the biochemical break-

115

down of the fungal elements. This manifests as a boggy mass or swelling in the scalp – a *kerion* – and indicates that the body is getting rid of the infection itself. The kerion is sterile. It will not grow any fungus. Hair loss occurs in the kerion and may occur in the areas of fungus infection, but the hair will grow back after resolution of the *Tinea capitis*.

A few of the species causing scalp ringworm fluoresce when exposed to Wood's light in a dark room. The light source is a long ultraviolet wavelength filtered through a special glass (Barium silicate with 9 per cent nickel oxide). Wood's light is compact and can be readily carried from place to place. Therefore, it is a rapid screening method for use in schools and institutions. Specific diagnosis is made by examining infected hairs under the microscope and by fungal culture.

Treatment consists of a course of oral griseofulvin, combined with topical antifungals and frequent shampoos. Secondary bacterial infection may be present. In this case, systemic antibiotics will need to be prescribed.

In certain parts of the world, the Middle East and Greenland in particular, a virulent type of fungus infection exists, which causes heavy white crusts around hairs. If left untreated, scarring and permanent hair loss results. This disease, favus – also known by the misnomer Norwegian scabies – is fortunately not indigenous to Great Britain and is rarely seen in this country.

Ringworm of the Feet (*Tinea pedis*)

Feet are commonly infected with either an acute or chronic fungus infection. In the acute stage vesicles of 2 to 3 mm appear on the soles, usually on the instep. This may resolve spontaneously, or progress to the chronic stage when left untreated.

Dry, scaly soles, often with some redness, characterize the chronic stage. The scaly redness may extend up around the heels and sides of the feet. Moist, white, macerated skin may be present in the toe webs. The chronic state may persist for years, waxing and waning in severity. In time, the toenails may become involved. The nail plate becomes thick and yellow with crusting beneath it that often lifts the nail up from its nail bed.

Frequent immersion of the feet in water, either through heavy sweating or because of one's occupation, predisposes to infection. The disease is common in hot, humid climates. Soldiers assigned to the tropics and required to march in heavy boots are, especially, susceptible. They call the infection, 'jungle rot'. Athletes are also at higher risk. Hence, the name, athlete's foot.

Treatment. The feet must be kept dry. This helps in prevention and helps in cure. Wear shoes that allow ventilation. Tennis shoes, sneakers, boots make feet sweat; their use should be limited. If you have to wear them, remove them when you come home – wash your feet, pat dry and apply a foot powder. Do not neglect the toe webs. They should be dried well and powder applied.

Aluminium acetate soaks (Burrows solution), 1:20 dilution, for ten or fifteen minutes twice daily help decrease sweating and dry the vesicles of the acute stage.

Prescription antifungal creams (clotrimazole, miconazole) will help clear the acute infection and some chronic infections. The latter often requires oral griseofulvin. Even then it is usually hard to cure and may recur once the medicine is stopped. Toenail infections are especially hard to cure. The nails may need to be removed and you will have to take long-term griseofulvin for months. If you cannot practise preventive measures, or you wear old infected shoes, or walk barefoot in contaminated areas, the infection will return. Some people learn to live with their chronic infection if it is not causing any serious problems.

Ringworm of the Hand (*Tinea manuum*)

Infection of the hands is infrequent and, usually, secondary to a long-standing infection of the feet. Typically one hand becomes involved, with dry peeling and non-itchy redness of the palm. Involvement of both hands is uncommon. Finger-nails may be involved with or without evident palmar changes. The tops of the hands are not involved with redness and scaling.

Contributing factors are frequent immersion in water, sweating and repeated contact to an infected source.

Treatment is similar to that for the feet, and has to include the feet when they are the source of the problem.

Ringworm of the groin (*Tinea cruris*)

Moist, scaly red or tan oval patches occur in the groin where there is sweating, friction and occlusion of the area by heavy clothes. The patches often show a sharp border with vesicles in the early active stage. Later, they become drier, scaly and change colour from red to brown.

The condition is common in men who sweat profusely and wear tight 'jockey' shorts. Obesity also contributes to the problem.

Microscopic examination of scrapings from the active border should help establish a definitive diagnosis.

Treatment. Although not difficult to treat, it may be hard to cure – coming and going over many years. Keeping the groin dry with antifungal powders and wearing loose under-pants, preferably cotton, will aid in both prevention and treatment. Topical antifungal medications usually clear the problem. Occasionally a short course of oral griseofulvin is required.

Ringworm of the Beard (*Tinea barbae*)

An uncommon fungus, *Tricophyton verrucosum* may cause an infection in bearded men who work with horses. Men who do not work with horses are less likely to contact the organism.

Scaly papules and crusts occur around the beard hairs. There may be secondary bacterial infection too. Diagnosis is by history, scraping and culture.

Treatment of choice is oral griseofulvin and adjunctive topicals.

Common Fungus Species Causing Ringworm

Trichophytum mentagrophytes and *Trichophytum rubrum* are more likely to produce feet and hand infections. *T. rubrum* presents as a more dry, scaly involvement than does *T. mentagrophytes* which is apt to cause a more vesicular infection. The *Microsporum* species – *canis* and *audoinii* – are more likely to cause body infections. However, none of the aforementioned species is exclusive to an area, and may cause infections on the scalp or body. Their prevalence also varies in geographic areas. In one city, a certain species may more often cause a scalp infection, while a different species will be the culprit in a second city.

Epidermophyton floccosum usually causes groin infections.

The species can be identified only by culture, since each has distinctive characteristics. On skin scraping examination, they all look alike microscopically.

If you want detailed and complete information on the organisms, a mycology text will provide this for you.

TINEA VERSICOLOR

An innocuous fungus, *Malessia furfur* infects the top scaly layer (stratum corneum), causing changes that draw one's attention to the skin. There are no symptoms. Versicolour, as the name suggests, means a variety of colours. Oval white to tan, sometimes yellowish or pink, spots of about 5 mm in diameter appear on preferred sites – chest, back, shoulders, upper arms and the sides of the neck. They are numerous and have a fine surface scaling. The colour change will make you wonder what is happening to your skin and prompt you to see a doctor.

Occasionally, underlying factors, e.g. diabetes or long-term oral steroids, may predispose to this infection. However, the condition is relatively common among vigorous, young healthy adults. It is passed from person to person through close, intimate contact, or from contaminated object to person. Sweating and chafing from tight, rough clothing will contribute to the infection.

The dermatologist should easily make the diagnosis by the distinctive appearance of the skin. Sometimes, there may be confusion with *pityriasis alba* (see p. 112), or an atypical *pityriasis rosea* (see p. 113). A microscopic examination of skin scrapings will readily show the difference. The doctor will see the typical 'spaghetti and meat balls' appearance of the hyphae and spores that characterize the causative organism.

Treatment. Since the organism is easily shed into clothes, bedding and furnishings, reinfection is common. Therefore, eradication of the infection may be difficult. At the time of treatment, you should also wash or clean things with which you are in close contact in order to minimize reinfection.

Therapy is basically aimed at peeling off the infected superficial skin layer. Good results are obtained with application of one per cent selenium sulphide in a water-miscible ointment base, which is applied three times weekly and left on for ten minutes, then washed off. Selenium shampoo can be substituted. Other treatments are 20 per cent aqueous sodium hyposulphite twice daily for six to eight weeks, or salicylic acid and sulphur ointment BPC.

INTERTRIGO

Any crease or body fold can develop a skin irritation and secondary infection from sweat and chafing. Frequent areas of involvement are the groin, armpits, the fold under large breasts, and the crease under a pendulous abdominal fat pad in obese people.

After the skin is irritated, opportunistic surface yeast and bacteria move in to create an exudative red shiny rash.

Treatment is uncomplicated. An anti-yeast, anti-bacterial combination cream with hydrocortisone (trimovate) is quite effective when applied three times daily. Adjunctive therapy is aimed at keeping the area clean with gentle washing, and dry with anti-fungal powder.

Contributing problems such as obesity, poor nutrition or diabetes mellitus should be corrected or controlled.

YEAST INFECTIONS (THRUSH, CANDIDIASIS, MONILIASIS)

Candida albicans, a yeast fungus, may cause infections of the skin. It is not part of the natural skin flora (other yeast organisms are), but is acquired from contact with carriers and contaminated objects. The organism is an opportunist, taking ready advantage of either an irritated or dermatitic local skin condition or of compromised general health.

In skin folds, chafing, sweating and a pre-existing rash, such as seborrhoeic dermatitis, predispose to candidiasis. It is often a component of nappy rash.

It may occur secondary to the systemic effects of broad spectrum antibiotics (tetracyclines), steroids, chemotherapy, poor nutrition, lymphomas, immune deficiency states or diabetes mellitus. When treating for candidiasis, the doctor should always inquire about your general health.

121

The typical infection, located in creases, shows a white exudate over a moist shiny red inflammation. At the periphery, flaccid pustules about 3 to 4 mm across are present. They and the exudate are full of yeast organisms. Common intertrigo may have an overgrowth of Candida. Scrapings examined microscopically will show an abundance of circular spores but no hyphae. This is diagnostic and separates the yeast fungus from the hyphae fungi of ringworm and the spore and hyphae fungus of *Tinea versicolor*. In contrast to the ringworm fungi, a culture of Candida grows rapidly – showing white yeasty growth in four to five days.

When the mouth is infected, it shows white exudative patches, 'thrush', on the tongue and elsewhere. Vaginal infections are relatively common, more so with the intake of tetracyclines.

People who immerse their hands in dirty water a lot – housewives, housemaids, waiters and waitresses – may develop a yeast infection between the finger web, or of the fingernail (or nails). At times, the skin round the nail may get infected and become swollen and painful. This is known as a paronychion.

Treatment consists of keeping the hands dry and soaking with a 1:20 dilution of Burrow's or aluminium acetate solution, and applying anti-fungal topicals, either nystatin or amphotericin.

Nystatin preparations are the ones of choice in the treatment of uncomplicated yeast infections. Often Candida intertrigo has an accompanying bacterial component, or common intertrigo is infected with secondary Candida. Then a triple combination topical (trimovate) is in order.

Every attempt should be made to correct a condition predisposing to candidiasis. Broad spectrum antibiotics or steroids should be stopped; poor nutrition should be corrected, etcetera.

Candidal infections unresponsive to topical care may

respond with good results to ketoconazole orally. However, liver toxicity has been reported, and the medication should be prescribed judiciously by the doctor.

SEBORRHOEIC DERMATITIS

Dermatologists often lump this quite common skin disease with the constitutional group of dermatitis – atopic dermatitis, discoid dermatitis and so on. However, there is little similarity clinically or microscopically. In fact, there seems to be a closer relationship between seborrhoeic dermatitis and psoriasis, than with any other skin disease. This will be discussed later.

'Seborrhoeic' means greasy and refers to sebum, the oily substance secreted by the oil (sebaceous) glands. These glands are prevalent on the face, upper back and upper chest. Since seborrhoeic dermatitis presents as reddish patches with a soft, greasy-feeling scale in oily areas of the body, early dermatologists, naturally, assumed the condition had something to do with the oil gland, and that the scale was sebum.

Advances in research techniques have since shown that the greasy encrustation is not sebum, but keratin, the scaly component of the epidermis, and that the keratin itself accounts for the greasy scale. Furthermore, increased secretion of oil glands has not been demonstrated in seborrhoeic dermatitis. Therefore, an association has not been established between the two.

However, this does not answer the question of the greasy scale, since keratin scales in the dermatitis/eczema group are dry, even when the rash is located in the same sites where seborrhoeic dermatitis might erupt. Therefore, it is believed that the oil glands do play some as yet undefined role in seborrhoeic dermatitis. Other reasons for this are as follows.

Seborrhoeic dermatitis occurs most often in non-hairy and

123

hairy areas where there is an abundance of oil glands. Hair has associated oil glands whose ducts empty into the hair's pore. Furthermore, seborrhoeic dermatitis appears at times of life when the sebaceous glands are physiologically active, i.e. infancy, adolescence and adulthood. There is speculation that a mother's hormones during gestation are somehow responsible for sebaceous gland activity during infancy. Thus the infant may develop seborrhoeic dermatitis as soft, greasy scales of the scalp (cradle cap), or as redness and scaling of the cheeks or nappy area.

Following infancy, there is little sebaceous gland activity until adolescence, when hormonal changes stimulate the oil glands. Then seborrhoeic dermatitis manifests itself again.

Most of us have a mild form of seborrhoeic dermatitis at some time during our lives. This is common dandruff. Usually, the problem is no more than that, but in some individuals it progresses to form superficial red patches with heavier scaling. This can extend to involve the ears, external ear canal, eyebrows, forehead and flush areas of the face. They will show a fine flaking on pinkish skin. The nose and the folds from the nose to the lips can be involved, as can the eyelids. The eyelid margins may get red and scaly, and there may be a discharge at the corners of the eye. The eyelid involvement is called 'seborrhoeic blepharitis'. Occasionally, the whites of the eye become irritated.

In men, a beard may hide patches of rash as can a hairy chest, and back.

The initial lesions are flat, red, slightly scaling ovals of about 4 mm to 1 cm across. They can combine into larger lesions, characterized by the yellowish soft scale. On the scalp and face the borders are usually indistinct, while on the trunk, over the sternum and between the shoulder blades, the borders are sharply defined.

By and large the lesions are dry, except when they occur in flexures and folds where sweat and friction make them moist and macerated. Seborrhoeic dermatitis, then, has a wet, reddish brown appearance and the scale is not so obvious. Secondary infection with bacteria and yeast may complicate the eruption and create a florid intertrigo. Then it may be hard for the doctor to ascertain the original problem.

How to Tell Seborrhoeic Dermatitis from the Eczema Group

The eczemas itch; seborrhoeic dermatitis, usually, does not. Also, eczemas have an inherent blistering component; seborrhoeic dermatitis does not. Furthermore, lesions of the latter are red and have a sharper, more distinct border than lesions of eczema.

Distribution is also a distinguishing feature. Eczemas can occur anywhere on the body, while seborrhoeic dermatitis primarily affects the oily, hairy and intertriginous regions.

When chronic dermatitis localizes to the scalp, it may be difficult to tell from a thick plaque of seborrhoeic dermatitis. Although seborrhoea normally does not itch, it may when there is heavy scalp involvement. To help make the diagnosis, a small skin biopsy, known as a punch biopsy, can be done, and the specimen prepared on a glass slide and diagnosed microscopically.

If anything, seborrhoeic dermatitis bears similarities to psoriasis. This condition will be discussed in the next chapter. The two may co-exist, with seborrhoeic dermatitis on the scalp seeming to merge into a thicker plaque of psoriasis. Sometimes, a greasy-looking patch is thicker than usual and resistant to the milder treatment needed for seborrhoea. These lesions are not quite seborrhoeic dermatitis, nor quite psoriasis. Doctors often straddle the fence and call them sebopsoriasis – in effect, a seborrhoeic dermatitis evolving into psoriasis.

Microscopic features also point to an association, since skin biopsies of sebopsoriasis will show features suggestive, if not totally diagnostic, of psoriasis. The importance of these similarities is unclear.

Origin and Associated Factors

We have much information about the appearance of seborrhoeic dermatitis, the extent of involvement, and how to treat it, but precious little is known about the origin of this common condition. Genetic constitution plays a role in determining whether or not a person develops seborrhoeic dermatitis. Many of us have oily skin, but we do not all get red, scaly rashes around our nose and in our eyebrows.

At one time, a superficial yeast fungus, found profusely in scalp lesions, was thought to contribute to seborrhoeic dermatitis. Advertisements of twenty years ago or more proclaimed *Pityrosporum ovale* (pronounced pity-ross-pore-um O-val-ee) as the cause of dandruff. A drawing of a large microscopic lens with fungal spores and S-shaped threads (hyphae) enlarged a hundred-fold depicted what the creatures were really like. This, plus the horror-stricken face of a victim as he stared at dandruff flakes on his shoulder, was calculated to drive the consumer to the nearest chemist for the advertised shampoo.

Later, dermatologists dismissed *P. ovale* as a causative agent. It was considered a normal resident in scalps of many people, with and without seborrhoea – one that thrived in greasy scales without contributing to their origin.

Recently, however, dermatologists have, experimentally, shown that the use of oral ketoconazole decreases *P. ovale* and improves seborrhoeic dermatitis. Topical anti-fungal lotions will do the same. Thus, the belief that *P. ovale* contributes to the cause of seborrhoeic dermatitis has come full circle, although the precise nature of its role remains to be determined.

Seborrhoeic dermatitis may be associated with certain diseases. Some, such as Parkinsonism and epilepsy, are neurological in origin. Others, like adult diabetes, have a hormonal basis. Skin diseases in which there is an oily skin – acne and rosacea or adult acne – often have associated seborrhoea.

Conditions that cause increased sweating and flushing will encourage seborrhoeic dermatitis. Therefore, emotional stress is frequently a contributing factor, often the most important one. People who blush easily may develop a facial rash in the blush areas.

Diet also plays a role. Alcoholism commonly exacerbates the condition. A high fat intake with ingestion of large amounts of dairy products, bacon or other fatty meats and peanut butter, will contribute to the problem, so can stimulants – coffee, tea, chocolate, drugs (cocaine).

Prevention and Treatment

Several things can be done to prevent or diminish the eruption of seborrhoeic dermatitis. Often its presence is the result of neglecting your health.

Diminish emotional tension as much as is humanly possible (see Chapter 9). Avoid or minimize alcohol and stimulants. If you are overweight, see your doctor about a weight reduction programme, and make sure the doctor does a test to rule out latent diabetes. Keep skin folds dry – pat the area well with a soft towel and apply a dusting powder.

Do not neglect your face and scalp if you have a tendency towards oiliness. Shampoo your hair three times weekly, daily if needed, with one of the tar or salicylic acid shampoos. You can buy them without prescription from the chemist. Wash your face about twice daily. Simple measures like this can prevent a red, scaly outbreak.

If the condition becomes full blown, treatment is straightforward. Use daily anti-dandruff shampoos until the dermatitis improves. An over-the-counter salicylic acid cream may get rid of the rash on the trunk and ears. However, it may irritate the face, so do not use it there. And do not use it in creases where it may accumulate to cause irritation.

Affected intertriginous areas need to be dried with soothing astringent compresses (Burrows solution 1:20 dilution). Topical corticosteroids combined with anti-infectives are effective. When there is a concomitant yeast infection, a combination cream such as trimovate is good to use.

In hairy or intertriginous areas uncomplicated by infection, steroid lotions, Class III or IV potency, should be used. Mild hydrocortisone creams, not ointments, applied two or three times a day to the face and other non-hairy areas should clear most seborrhoeic dermatitis.

A low-fat diet is advised. Such a diet is healthful and will improve your general well-being, even if a direct correlation with your rash is not readily apparent.

Chapter Seven

PSORIASIS

A discussion of seborrhoeic dermatitis leads us, naturally, to a discussion of psoriasis – a skin affliction which ranks along with seborrhoeic dermatitis, the dermatitis group and drug reactions, as one of the most common. Two per cent of the population has the disease. Psoriasis can arise at any age, but is most common in young adults. The mean age is twenty-seven, but the spectrum ranges from infancy to the elderly. Men and women are equally affected.

Insensitive people make jokes about the 'heartbreak of psoriasis'. However, if you have psoriasis, you know it is not a laughing matter.

More than the skin is involved in this malady. In fact, it is not accurate to think of psoriasis as just a skin disease. Rather, the typical red plaques are a manifestation of aberrant immunological and cellular changes going on within the body.

Currently, much research is being done on psoriasis. Information is accumulating that supports a genetic link. Genetic markers have been identified, which are associated with a high risk for developing psoriasis. Immunological abnormalities have been discovered, not only in patients, but in close relatives who do not show the disease.

Studies of the epidermis reveal a rapid turnover of the skin cell cycle from its origin in the basal layer to formation of the scaly stratum corneum. This means psoriatic epidermis forms at a much faster rate than normal skin. The latter takes about twenty-eight days to replace itself. In psoriasis, the time is reduced to about three days.

As information mounts, it becomes evident that psoriasis is a condition of much complexity. Discoveries have come as isolated pieces of knowledge. Medical researchers are something like the blind man groping at an elephant – first he discovers the foot, then the ear, next the tail. Before our elephant is identified, important parts have yet to be revealed. Only then will we have a complete understanding of the mechanisms behind the clinical disease.

What Does It Look Like?

The psoriatic plaque is a typical and characteristic lesion (see Fig. 9B). It is red, sharply demarcated at the borders and raised about 1 to 4 mm above the surface with a silvery white (frosty-looking) adherent scale. In the moist (flexual, fold, genital) areas, or with acute psoriasis, the scale may not be evident. The size of the plaque can vary from a couple of millimetres to several centimetres in size.

Early or more acute psoriasis often presents with multiple small red lesions of about 4 to 8 mm across, distributed over the trunk and limbs. The scale, although present, will not be as marked as in larger plaques.

Psoriasis presents in a variety of forms and patterns, which are given descriptive names. The sudden, acute type, mentioned above, is the 'guttate' type. The 'plaque' form is more chronic and may have a 'gyrate' pattern, and so on. The clinical manifestation may be acute or chronic, with one lesion, or many lesions. The course may be of short duration, or long, with remissions and relapses. The nails and scalp may be involved too.

Plaques, typically, appear in pressure areas, e.g. over elbows and knees. This extensor preference contrasts with the flexural involvement of atopic dermatitis.

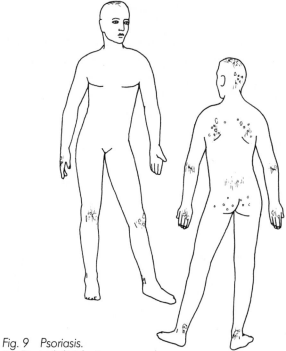

Fig. 9 Psoriasis.
A Typical distribution:
   Lesions are primarily on extensor surfaces and pressure areas.
   Compare to atopic dermatitis, Fig. 6.
B Hand: Typical plaques with nail involvement.

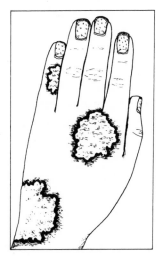

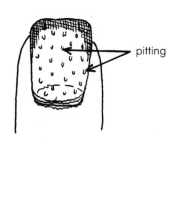

pitting

Pustular psoriasis, a rare, severe form, may erupt as a result of sudden withdrawal of steroids for treatment of a pre-existing psoriasis, or possibly for treatment of another condition in a patient with psoriasis. As a rule, therefore, systemic steroids are not advised in psoriatic treatment.

A pre-existing psoriasis, especially of the guttate variety, may erupt into pustular psoriasis, if sensitized by topical medications or treated too vigorously with ultraviolet light and tar.

Large areas of the body are involved in pustular psoriasis. Patients are sick, have a fever and require hospitalization. With a better understanding of psoriasis and modern methods of treatment, this complication is fortunately very infrequent.

Sterile pustules, whether evident clinically or only microscopically, are an identifying feature of psoriasis. They may occur in localized psoriasis, especially of the acute type. A pustular form of the palms and soles exists too. Chronic dry plaques will contain microscopic pustules. These micro-abscesses, collections of white cells called *neutrophils*, are a diagnostic feature when a processed skin biopsy is viewed under the microscope. They are found in the thickened scaly top layer (stratum corneum) of the epidermis.

In the dermatitis group, vesicles within the epidermis contain tissue fluid (oedema). In psoriasis there is no oedema. Instead, small collections of neutrophils gather, and travel through the epidermis to form micro-abscesses. The significance of these tiny pustules and their relationship to the psoriatic process remain unclear.

Finger- and toe-nails may be affected. Early changes show pitting of the nail plate. Later the nail may thicken, become yellow and crumbly. To all outward appearances, it resembles a fungus infection. Microscopic examination of nail scrapings and cultures of the affected nail may be necessary in order to make the differentiation. Sometimes, even that will not give the answer, and the doctor has to rely on his or her clinical judgement. When the psoriasis clears, the nails should gradually return to normal. At times, a nail will come off and a new one will grow in its place.

In about 10 per cent of patients, *arthritis* is part of psoriasis. Some studies report an incidence as high as 20 per cent. It can be a minor problem or major complication with pain, swelling and eventual deformity. Clinically, it affects the same joints as rheumatoid arthritis. But the biochemical changes present in rheumatoid arthritis are not present in psoriatic arthritis. Therefore, these arthritic conditions are assumed to be different from each other. The treatment of psoriatic arthritis, although similar to rheumatoid arthritis, has to be considered in the context of the psoriatic problem in general.

Is There Any Chance of Confusing Psoriasis with the Eczemas?

The answer to this question should be, 'Highly unlikely'. Psoriasis seldom itches and is not exudative, in contrast to dermatitis. Unlike atopic dermatitis, it affects, primarily, extensor areas (elbows, knees, sacrum) (see Fig. 9A), while the former affects the flexor regions (see Fig. 6).

Occasionally, a chronic dermatitis will localize over the knees or elbows, and will be hard to distinguish from psoriasis. Whether it itches or not cannot be used to make the distinction, since itching is a subjective response. While some people itch, others will not. There are patients who complain of severe itching with psoriasis. Anything on their skin seems to provoke an itch-scratch cycle. When there is doubt about diagnosis, a small skin biopsy usually helps to make the distinction.

Two interesting clinical observations regarding psoriasis help to distinguish it further from dermatitis, as well as other common skin eruptions. The 'Auspitz sign', named after the observant doctor who first described it, is one of them. When the white adherent scale is scraped away, pinpoint surface bleeding spots develop. They coincide with microscopic capillaries that are close to the surface, and no doubt account for the redness of psoriasis. This sign is specific for psoriasis and a helpful diagnostic tool.

The second observation, the Koebner phenomenon, named after another astute physician, is an interesting characteristic of psoriasis. In active psoriasis, if the skin is scratched, bruised, cut or damaged in any way, psoriatic lesions will appear at the site of injury. For example, after abdominal surgery, one is likely to get psoriasis in the surgery line. In early psoriasis, the skin apparently is reactive and has the potential to develop psoriasis anywhere on the surface.

This phenomenon does not occur in dermatitis. However, it is not unique to psoriasis. A few, uncommon, unrelated skin diseases may show the Koebner phenomenon. *Lichen planus* (p. 100) is one of them.

For a discussion of seborrhoeic dermatitis and psoriasis, see Chapter 6.

What Can be Done about Psoriasis?

Management should be individualized to the needs of the patient. If you have psoriasis, you may have one plaque, or several, or the psoriasis may be confined to your scalp and nails, and so on. All this will determine the approach to your treatment.

Your attitude is important. Worry and frustration about your plight will only make psoriasis worse. Dr Farber, who heads a psoriasis research programme at Stanford University in the US, has done studies showing that extreme emotional stress makes psoriasis worse in 40 per cent of the cases.

Be positive and hopeful. Yours is not a life and death matter. Retain your sense of humour – remind your friends that your scales are not contagious, and remember the lesions resolve without scarring. Practise methods of relaxation to diminish stress (see Chapter 9).

Treatment

Several methods are currently available. Some are old methods, others are newer modifications of them, and others are due to recent advances in the field. All improve psoriasis – some faster than others. The right approach needs to be selected for you.

Sunlight alone will improve most psoriasis. Gradual exposure, permitting the skin to tan rather than burn, is important. A sunburn can cause enough skin damage to worsen psoriasis, especially in the early stage. Guttate psoriasis is more likely to react like this.

Dithranol in Lasser's paste (zinc and salicylic acid paste) is a common treatment, in Britain, for chronic plaque psoriasis. Results have been good, but dithranol has the disadvantage of staining, and can cause irritation. Sensitive areas (face and flexural folds) should be treated carefully with weak concentrations, or not at all with this preparation.

A single plaque, or a few plaques, can be adequately treated with coal tar preparations with or without ultraviolet light. The latter, however, improves the action of coal tar substantially. This combination is the basis for an effective treatment regimen – the Goeckerman Technique.

Goeckerman Technique. Coal tar is applied to plaques. Twelve to twenty-four hours later it is removed with mineral oil and ultraviolet light is administered. The treatment is repeated daily or three to four times weekly. Since the routine is messy and time-consuming, patients are often hospitalized to facilitate treatment. The response is good. Plaques clear in about three weeks and remission lasts for several months. But remember tar can irritate or sensitize.

The *Ingram method* is a modification of the Goeckerman regimen, which is more effective and produces longer remissions. Hospitalization is usually necessary because of the time-consuming and messy aspects of the treatment, although with experienced staff outpatient treatment can also be done. The method is as follows: you will take daily tar baths, followed by ultraviolet light three times weekly after the baths; dithranol in Lasser's paste or in a mixture of paraffin is applied to your lesions, starting with a 0.05 per cent concentration and working up to 0.5 per cent, if needed. You are then covered with tubinette (a tubular gauze which keeps the paste in place) for twenty-four hours. Next, you are unwrapped and the dithranol removed with liquid paraffin or arachis (peanut) oil. The treatments are repeated. Clearing occurs in two or three weeks and remission lasts for months.

A note of caution. On the face and genital area, dithranol should be applied in low concentrations, if at all. Care must be taken not to smear the paste away from the lesions, as burning and irritation can occur.

Corticosteroids. Systemic steroids should not be taken for psoriasis. They will quickly clear you, but you may find yourself in the proverbial 'tiger by the tail' situation. When the steroids are discontinued, you may rebound to become worse than you were in the beginning. You may even develop an acute extensive pustular psoriasis, or an erythroderma (the red skin of a generalized exfoliative dermatitis; see p. 31). For control, you will be forced back on the steroids to suffer the consequences of their long-term effects.

Topical steroids are highly effective and are frequently used. The more potent fluorinated ones are the common choice. However, on the face and flexures, weaker strengths should be applied. (See Chapter 10.)

The plaques should clear rapidly with topical treatment. Again there is a possibility of 'rebound' when the steroid preparation is stopped. The best approach is to wean yourself off the steroids. Apply the medication less frequently – every other day or third day when your skin improves. Or ask your doctor for a weaker steroid which can be substituted for the stronger one, and gradually stopped.

Methotrexate, a chemotherapeutic agent used in cancer therapy, is very effective in the treatment of psoriasis, but can have serious consequences. Liver scarring with liver failure and death have been reported. Bone marrow depression with decreased white blood cell formation may be a problem. Also, abnormalities can occur in new and rapidly growing tissue. Women in the child-bearing years have to be very carefully screened. In pregnancy, the foetus would be irreparably damaged by this drug.

Because of the side-effects, strict guidelines are used in the selection of patients for treatment. Only healthy, non-pregnant individuals with severe, resistant psoriasis that interferes with personal life and work are candidates. Before starting treatment, a thorough physical examination should always be done. An oral dose of methotrexate, based on the body weight, is taken weekly with good results. Often, the remission is not as prolonged as with the Goeckerman or Ingram methods. Maintenance doses, with close monitoring of liver and blood can be given.

PUVA, a recently developed method, has produced good therapeutic results. The 'P' stands for psoralen and 'UVA' stands for long wave length ultraviolet A light.

As I discussed in the section on photodermatitis, the psoralens are strong photosensitizers. They exist in certain plants as furocoumarin compounds, complex chemicals. Psoralens are either extracted from these plants or synthesized in the laboratory. 8-methoxypsoralen, the drug used in PUVA therapy, is extracted from plants of the Umbelliferae (fennel, dill) family.

If you receive PUVA therapy, the treatment goes like this: First you will take tablets of 8-methoxypsoralen (the dose will be determined by your weight), and two hours later you will receive a dose of long wave UV light, known as UVA. At this particular time, the concentration of psoralen in your blood is at its maximum peak. The psoralen, activated by the UV light, forms a substance which inhibits DNA synthesis and cell division. Rapidly dividing cells, such as in psoriatic plaques, are particularly sensitive to this inhibition.

The UV treatment is administered in a cabinet containing UV-emitting fluorescent tubing. Initial exposures are determined by your skin type. The time of exposure increases with subsequent exposures, as your skin tans and develops more UV light tolerance.

Treatment continues two to four times weekly until the lesions clear. The average number of treatments is fifteen. A good result occurs in most cases of psoriasis. Chronic plaques and pustular lesions of the palms and soles are most responsive.

Initial reaction to PUVA treatment was very enthusiastic, since it has several advantages over other methods. It is very effective, easy to give, eliminates the mess of ointments and pastes and the nuisance of wraps, and can be given on an outpatient basis.

However, as with any newer treatment, enthusiasm should be checked until the long-term effects of such treatment become available. Studies give evidence of the need for caution. Psoralens potentiate the effects of UV light on the entire skin, not solely in plaques. Accelerated changes of ageing, as occur with excess sun exposure, have been demonstrated in treated patients. Whether these changes will eventually lead to an increase in skin cancers remains to be seen. But it seems that such patients are at greater risk.

There is also experimental evidence that psoralens cause mutations (abnormal changes in the cell nucleus) in bacteria and mammalian cells while they are kept in the dark. Exposure to ultraviolet light markedly increases this mutagenic effect. With PUVA treatment, the mutagenic potential of psoralen may be transferred to human cells to further increase the risk of cancer. Time will decide if this will be the case.

Finally, PUVA therapy requires a special cabinet and special lights which are expensive to install. Many hospital clinics cannot afford this form of therapy. Therefore the treatment may not be available to you.

A new drug, *Tigason*, a derivative of vitamin A, can be given in small doses alone or with PUVA therapy. The consequences are beneficial. Tigason increases ultraviolet activity. The light dose is then cut in half. The drug also helps PUVA treatment clear unresponsive plaques. Few side effects have thus far been imputed to it.

Experimental studies with another vitamin A derivative, *etretinate*, are showing its value in psoriatic treatment, especially in chronic plaques, but the drug has yet to be released for general use.

All sorts of *diets* have been tried in psoriasis. One of them, a three-week turkey diet, deprived the body of an essential nutrient. The psoriasis cleared, but patients could not remain on the diet without the danger of malnutrition and eventual death. The answer does not lie in special diets. A sensible, well-balanced diet should suffice.

Localized areas will need special attention. The scalp, when involved, should be washed daily with tar shampoos, and steroid lotions rubbed into it two or three times a day. The treatment is like that for seborrhoeic dermatitis, but much more intense.

Nail changes are difficult to treat. Fortunately, they should improve when the general problem improves. If the psoriasis mainly affects the nails, then specific attention will have to be directed towards them.

Sunlight and relaxation help improve psoriatic nails. Strong topical steroids can be applied under occlusion with relatively good results. Some doctors inject intralesional steroids into the base of the nail, since the nail arises from cells in this area. I certainly do not advise injections with a needle – they are too painful. But a dermojet, which injects a squirt of medicine into the skin under pressure, is relatively painless.

Flexures and folds will need to be dried first with mild soap washes or astringent compresses (normal saline, aluminium acetate). After this, steroids of moderate to mild potency should be applied. Other preparations (tar, dithranol) can be irritants in these areas and should be avoided.

Chapter Eight

A COUPLE
OF LOOK-ALIKES

Two skin diseases – one rare, the other common – may be mistaken for acute dermatitis and, occasionally, for each other. One, dermatitis herpetiformis (DH for simplicity) is genetically determined. The other, scabies, is a common infestation of the skin, which produces very itchy vesicles and may either provoke or complicate dermatitis.

It is worth spending some time on them.

DERMATITIS HERPETIFORMIS (DH)

Severe itching and the appearance of small vesicles and wheals might make us think of a contact dermatitis to sprays, clothing or detergents. But DH is nothing of the kind.

If we look closely, we will notice that the distribution of the lesions is atypical for a dermatitis. Also, although the eruption at first looks as though it might be a contact dermatitis, we soon realize that the lesions are discrete and do not clump together into itchy, moist, scaly patches as does a contact dermatitis.

Tiny, red papules or vesicles on a red, urticarial base characterize the eruption. These appear in clusters, in a predominantly symmetrical distribution, involving the arms, knees and shoulders. The buttocks and the area between the shoulder blades are also commonly affected. Itching is fierce. Sometimes nothing is left of the lesions – they have all been replaced with scratch marks. At first the eruption might be mistaken for insect bites, but its chronicity and associated findings should dispel this idea. Occasionally, a few vesicles become large discrete blisters of about 1 cm in size.

The persistent discreteness of the lesions is very characteristic and distinguishes DH from eczema, which readily forms inflammatory patches.

The patient, typically a young man, will probably be thin and complain of diarrhoea and other digestive disturbances. He may also give a family history of similar problems.

A skin biopsy of one of the intact vesicles will give us the diagnosis. Examination of the prepared specimen microscopically will show the blister to be beneath the epidermis at its junction with the bottom layer of skin, the dermis. In dermatitis, the vesicle is within the epidermis. Furthermore, a special immunofluorescent test will show fluorescing granular deposit along the base of the vesicle in DH. This substance, identified as Immunoglobulin A, is present in the skin of patients with DH, but not in the skin of patients with eczema.

Immediately we know that there is an alteration in the patient's immune system in DH. We look further, examine the blood, and find circulating antibodies formed in reaction to the patient's own tissue (autoantibodies). Thus, it is possible that antibodies directed against the patient's own skin are causing the eruption. However, this is still conjecture.

An X-ray of the small bowel provides an interesting finding. Its convoluted lining is revealed as thin and flattened (atrophic). The changes are similar to those present in medical diseases where the small bowel is unable to absorb and/or digest nutrients. Eighty per cent of DH patients will show the small bowel abnormality.

There is an inability to digest gluten. When the patient is put on a gluten-free diet, the bowel problem corrects itself. If the diet can be maintained, the skin will eventually clear. However, the diet is basically indicated in the more severe cases, and most patients do not have to contend with it. The relationship between the bowel disorder, the immunological changes and the skin remains a mystery still.

Specific treatment is available for the skin lesions, however. Oral dapsone will control DH and needs to be taken continually in maintenance doses. Often the patient may prefer just to have his skin problem treated, and will tolerate the moderate bowel discomfort rather than have to eat the gluten-free diet. But a strict diet will lower the need for high doses of dapsone, or do away with the drug altogether.

The aim of the doctor should be to keep the patient on as low a maintenance dose as possible. Dapsone is a sulfone and one of a group of medicines that can cause serious side-effects. It is also a frequent cause of allergic drug eruptions.

SCABIES

A microscopic mite, *Sarcoptes scabei*, burrows under the top layer of the skin to cause severe itching and a tiny papule or vesicle at the entrance into its burrow.

The sites of penetration are, predominantly, the wrists and finger webs, but any flexures can be involved – the groin, axillary regions, bends of the elbows. Buttocks, nipples, genitals and waist-line are commonly involved too.

When you first see the vesicles, you might think you were exposed to a contactant that is irritating your skin. If you have atopic dermatitis, you might think it is beginning to flare up.

Sometimes the situation can become confusing. The secretions of the mite are irritating, and can provoke an eruption of atopic dermatitis in predisposed people. Therefore, the infestation can be obscured, even missed at first. And the topical steroids that the doctor will undoubtedly prescribe if he or she thinks you have dermatitis will make the infestation spread. The subsequent maddening itch and lack of improvement will drive you to the doctor again. Eventually, scabies will be considered as the underlying cause of your problem, and a search will be made for the confirmatory mite.

Scabies is very prevalent and occurs everywhere. One should think of it in any severe, unrelenting itching and scratching. Contagion is spread through close physical contact, e.g. a bed partner or other family members. Infected clothing, bedding and towels can also be sources of infestation.

Only the pregnant female mite is capable of causing infestation since the male dies soon after copulation. The pregnant female then burrows into the scaly stratum corneum of the epidermis. She does not get much deeper than this and lays her eggs inside the tiny burrow – two or three a day for about two months. After this she dies, no doubt exhausted by her labours. In two to four days, the eggs hatch into larvae which transform into nymphs and then into adults. The entire cycle then repeats itself.

The mite is not visible to the naked eye and the burrows are barely noticeable tiny threads. A search and close inspection – preferably with a magnifying lens – is the best way to spot the burrows. The best place to look for them is the finger webs.

The burrow is a slightly raised, sinuous grey-white thread about 5 to 15 mm in length. Visible at its terminus should be a dark 'dot', containing the mite. The 'dot' may actually be a small vesicle or pustule. Sometimes black specks, representing dirt or faeces, are present in the burrow.

With a pointed scalpel blade, the doctor can slit open the tunnel and scrape off the parasite, and transfer it to a glass

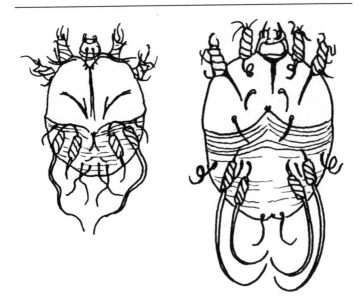

Fig. 10   The Scabies Mite – under the Microscope The scabies mite – under surface. The female is the larger of the two. The organism is oval, has four pairs of legs. By the naked eye, the mite will appear as a 'dot' when picked out of the skin by a pin. The male is not found, as he dies soon after copulation.

slide. A potassium hydroxide mount is then made. Examination under the microscope reveals the answer (see Fig. 10).

The burrows may be hard to find, especially if you bathe frequently and keep extra clean. Then a thorough search of your skin has to be made. Do not be ashamed or embarrassed if you do get scabies; it is not an infestation limited to the unwashed. It is highly contagious and can infect anyone from infants to the elderly, from lords to lorry drivers.

Relationship to Skin Allergies and Atopic Dermatitis

The skin reaction to the scabetic organism is a true allergic reaction. It takes place two to four weeks after the mite has penetrated the skin. In the meantime, you will have minimal, if any, reaction, and will not know you have been

145

infected. Should you get a second infection at some later date after you have been treated, you will react immediately with itching because your skin has already been sensitized by your first episode of infection.

However, reinfection is not common. The body probably develops an immunological resistance. All the mites entering the skin during the first infection are thought to stimulate the immune system, much like a series of immunization injections which then confer immunity.

The predominant component of the sensitization is itching. It is always worse at night. But other skin reactions occur too. A fine, reddish rash may appear, and patches of dermatitis often complicate the picture. Infection, secondary to scratching, may also be a problem.

As mentioned, a scabetic infection can play havoc in a person with atopic dermatitis. The irritating and sensitizing effects of the mite, not only create excruciating itch, but exacerbate the dermatitis. I have had patients come into my office – scratching, itching, pacing – unable to sit still.

Treatment

Once diagnosed, treatment is simple and curative. The following medications are prescribed topically: Eurax (crotamiton) cream or lotion, or one per cent gamma benzene hexachloride (quellada or Lorexane); 25 per cent benzyl benzoate emulsion can also be useful in treatment.

Crotamiton has the benefit of an anti-itch property. It is not as potent a scabeticide as gamma benzene hexachloride but is perfectly adequate, and does not have the potential for toxic reactions. On the other hand, gamma benzene hexachloride is readily absorbed through the skin and can cause toxic neurological changes in infants, and possibly in older children. Therefore, it should not be used for youngsters. In babies, 5 per cent precipitated sulphur in white paraffin (petrolatum) is safe and effective.

Crotamiton should be rubbed into the skin from neck to foot. Special attention needs to be given to folds and creases. The scalp, head and face do not need treatment, since they do not become infected.

Clothing, towels, bedding, any item in close contact with you should be washed thoroughly. Another treatment with crotamiton is done on the second day. Two days later, a cleansing bath is taken. All persons in close contact with you, whether they have actual signs of infection or not, should also be treated, since they may have the infection but not show signs of it as yet.

Some itching with a few papules may persist. This does not mean that infection continues, but that it takes the skin reaction a few days to subside. If the medication is applied correctly, the mite is killed quickly. For residual itching and papules, hydrocortisone cream should be effective.

If you have dry skin or atopic dermatitis, the scabies treatment may, occasionally, irritate your skin. You may continue to itch and scratch after treatment. And the resultant scratch papules may be mistaken for scabies. You will then believe that the scabies persists, and will, undoubtedly, do another treatment, which will further irritate your skin. The best thing to do is to give your skin a few days to recover from the initial treatment.

Emollient baths and hydrocortisone cream should relieve itch and irritation that results from the treatment. If symptoms continue to persist after seven or ten days, then a repeat scabies treatment can be considered.

Chapter Nine

STRESS

How many times have you heard phrases like, 'He makes my skin crawl', 'She rubs me up the wrong way', or 'Don't get hot under the collar'? These all associate skin reactions with emotions. Yet the speaker does not stop to think about the connection; he or she takes it for granted. Nevertheless, the psychic importance of the skin is once again established in the popular vernacular.

In medical practice, it is established through case histories. There are reports that 30 per cent of skin problems are directly psychological, and another 30 per cent are affected by the patient's psychological state.

Physiological Responses

Through complex neural and hormonal mechanisms, the skin reacts to stress. We have all seen the visible effects of emotion on the skin – the pallor of fear or anger, the blushing of embarrassment or shame, the sweat from nervous tension.

Our hearing and sight impinge on the brain's sensory cortex. It then sends impulses to an inner central part of our brain called the thalamus. From here, the impulses go through the spinal cord and travel through nerve fibres to end in a rich supply of fine autonomic nerve endings that exist beneath the epidermis. Certain biochemicals are now activated at these sites. They affect the cutaneous structures and blood vessels and therefore the state of the skin. (See below.)

More nerve pathways go to the brain from the skin than from any other organ. Nerve impulses, such as touch, pain, hot and cold sensations, also travel to the brain, and further impact on release of neurohumoural substances that affect the skin. Neurohumoural substances are biochemicals – e.g. acetylcholine, norepinephrine – released as a consequence of stimulation of the autonomic nervous system. The latter controls internal reactions, as opposed to external or muscular reactions which are controlled by voluntary motor nerve impulses, and does not concern us here.

In stressful situations, special hormones are released into the general circulation. In acute stress, the most important one is epinephrine (adrenalin) which comes from the central part of the adrenal gland. That organ sits like a cap over the kidney. Epinephrine makes the heart pound, turns the hands cold and sweaty, the mouth dry, and drives the blood pressure up, producing the typical 'fight or flight' reaction of fear and anger.

Chronic stress stimulates the secretion of corticosteroids. They are secreted by the outer part of the adrenal gland, the cortex. They have an effect on our immunological system and on many other biological processes (see Chapter 10).

Neural and hormonal induced physiological and biochemical responses cause specific cutaneous changes. Peripheral effects of vasoconstriction (narrowing of tiny arterioles with decreased blood flow), or of vasodilation (increased blood flow with increased skin temperature) affect flushing and sensations of heat and cold and therefore the skin's condition. Increased sweating that occurs on the palms, soles, in the genital/anal area and armpits affects those areas physically. And immune biochemical complexes may be deposited in the skin to affect it adversely.

It is evident that our emotions and body are intimately integrated, and stress, whether good or bad, can produce a skin reaction. One might break out in hives before receiving a trophy for some personal victory. And Masters and Johnson have reported a red, evanescent rash in couples during orgasm.

Skin Conditions Resulting Primarily from Psychological Problems

Self-inflicted skin injury. Many repressed, undesirable feelings can be displaced to the skin. Conditions with no organic basis will occur because of a patient's abuse of his integument. Individuals who do this are often deeply disturbed, sometimes psychotic.

The patient may burn or damage his skin to cause bizarre patterns of injury. Acids, lyes (caustic alkali preparations as found in oven cleaners), and cigarettes are some of the things used to do this.

Another manifestation of psychological illness is repetitive pulling or breaking off of one's hair. This is often seen in disturbed children and has been given the name, trichtillomania.

Parasitophobia (an obsessive fear of infestation) is more likely to be seen in an elderly patient who is convinced that some 'worm' or parasite resides in his skin. Itchy, dry skin may initiate the phobia. The patient will dig at the skin, peel bits of it off and place these in an envelope, which he will bring to the doctor, insisting that the bits of skin contained therein are bugs or worms. No one can persuade him otherwise. A patient who is challenged will, usually, get angry and leave, thinking that the doctor does not know anything. He is difficult to treat and often lives with his delusion.

Neurotic excoriation (nervous scratching). This condition is amenable to treatment. Anxiety, frustration or worry compels the patient, often a young woman, to scratch and dig at her skin. The sides of the arms, upper back and face are frequent targets. She will often recognize the psychological source of the problem. Support and understanding from the doctor and psychotherapy, if indicated, are very beneficial. Once the emotional distress clears, the picking compulsion goes away. Healing of the scratch marks can be facilitated with applications of a combination corticosteroid/anti-bacterial cream (see List 5, p. 163).

Nervous habits function in the release of emotional tension and can aggravate dermatitis. Biting nails and lips will irritate the skin, and exacerbate pre-existing rashes in these spots. Nail-biting may also introduce infections around the nail.

Licking of the lips, if continued repeatedly, will cause irritation and thickening of the lips. The skin around the lips may also become red and irritated resulting in a 'clown-like' appearance to the mouth. Children are more likely to have this habit than adults.

Once the habits cease, the skin will improve. Mild steroid creams or ointments will clear up the rash.

Skin Conditions Initiated or Exacerbated by Emotional Stress

I have discussed most of these, but mention them again to refresh your memory.

The dermatitis group (atopy, discoid dermatitis, hand dermatitis, ano-genital dermatitis, etc.), allergic reactions, urticaria and itching may all be stress related. To this can be added alopecia areata, a circular and temporary loss of scalp or beard hair which is sometimes associated with atopic dermatitis in young adults. Indeed, most skin eruptions can be affected by nervous stress which can make an existing problem worse, or cause the sudden appearance of a skin rash in a genetically predisposed person.

If you have a dermatitis, you may feel embarrassed and insecure. The sight of it on the visible parts of your body –

hands or face – will further add to despair and hamper improvement. The doctor's attitude is important. If he or she is relaxed, sympathetic and comfortable about touching your skin, you will feel better – less of an outcast.

The comfort and sympathy of someone close to you is obviously very important. But you should be your own best friend. Remember, the dermatitis is not contagious, will not leave scars, and will eventually go away.

Occasionally, an atypical form of localized dermatitis results from picking and scratching. This usually occurs on the legs of women and has been given the ungainly name of *prurigo nodularis*, meaning nodules arising as a result of itching and scratching. We may call them 'itch bumps'. They are about a centimetre or less in diameter and follow repeated scratching of a local eczema, a part of which thickens up into a 'knot'.

The skin in patients with this condition has a predilection for reacting in this way. In order to improve, one must stop scratching. Potent topical steroids (Class II or I – see Chapter 10) will resorb the nodules. Intralesional injections of steroids are useful, too.

Ano-genital dermatitis is usually eroticized and may be associated with emotional problems concerning sexuality. Plaques of dermatitis can occur on the scrotum, vulva and around the anal area. Of course physical factors, i.e. general health and local infections or infestations, should always be considered.

Minimizing Stress, Fostering Relaxation
'Relax', 'What's the rush?' These are common phrases thrown at us by well-meaning family and friends. The admonishment to relax is easier said than done. We cannot undo years of personality development and change our ways overnight. And some of us might be inherently highly strung and hyperactive. Besides, a certain degree of nervous stress

can be positive. It keeps us enthusiastic, energetic and excited about our life and work.

A proper balance needs to be maintained for good mental health. You do not want to be laid back to the point of lethargy and somnolence, nor do you want to be incapacitated by fear, anxiety, frustration, repression and other negative emotional responses.

Everyday life does not have to be fraught with heavy emotional crises to create nervous strain. The ordinary demands of job, family and your own demands of yourself will be enough to cause chronic anxiety. This in turn can aggravate your skin problem.

You should learn to eliminate bad stress and give yourself time to enjoy pleasurable moments. You should be your own best friend or best parent, and treat yourself accordingly. This means not being excessively demanding of yourself – allow the possibility of a mistake. If you make one, you will learn from it and next time do better.

If you are in a difficult work or personal relationship, get advice and counselling. It is available. Talking out something with a close friend, a spouse, being part of a support group, are all ways to help resolve personal problems. If your problems are complex and continuing, discuss them with your doctor who will be able to refer you to an appropriate therapist.

There are several simple accessible means by which you can relieve daily stress.

Learn to pace yourself. Plan ahead. Allow plenty of time in the morning to prepare for school or work without rushing. Leave in plenty of time to arrive at your destination. If you drive to work in heavy traffic, listen to soothing music rather than curse the driver in front of you. At traffic lights, sit back in your seat and relax. Do not hunch over the wheel with an impatient grip, as if you are waiting for the start of the big race.

Whether you are at work or busy at home, take fifteen minutes twice a day for relaxation. Sit in a comfortable chair – rocking chairs at home are nice – and let your mind wander to some pleasant spot, or meditate on a favourite poem or saying, or just let your eyes focus on some distant point. The goal is to allow your mind to drift without worrying about anything. Two or three slow deep breaths before you begin will help you get into the relaxation. People who practise transcendental meditation achieve the same type of relief from tension.

Muscle tension releasing exercises help in relaxation. They can be done at any time, during your relaxation periods, in the evening, or at night before you go to sleep. Begin by tightening your toes and feet, then relax them. Next, sequentially, tighten legs, buttocks, back and arm muscles. Finally, tighten all your muscles and relax. Hold the tension about two or three seconds. Breathe out when you tense your muscles and breathe in slowly when you relax them. If you have high blood pressure or heart disease, check with your doctor before attempting the tensing exercises.

Body massage is a pleasant way to relax and will improve intimacy between you and your partner.

Physical contact – warm, big hugs, hand holding, caressing and stroking should be encouraged between you and your partner, you and your children. If you do not have a partner or children, that is all right. Just give other family members or your friends hugs. It will not hurt them, and may pleasantly surprise them and you.

Affectionate body contact makes a person feel wanted, loved and fosters security and self-confidence. You will not feel unwanted because of your skin rash. If you have a partner, cuddling with him or her at night will encourage these feelings, too.

Take breaks away from your weekly routine. Plan at least one day a week for a pleasurable outing. If you have children, plan an evening away from them. Spend the time with your partner, or maybe you just need quiet time for yourself.

You may wish to take courses in relaxation. Many are available at nominal fees. Yoga, meditation, Chinese Tai Chi exercises, are all aimed at teaching relaxation. Check your borough's adult education list. You will find it in your local library.

Nervous tension may be improved with biofeedback methods. In this technique, instruments which record pulse and perspiration are attached to your fingers. A high pitched tone goes off when pulse and sweating rise with increase in nervous stress. You learn to control the stress by monitoring the tone. For some people this is too technical and impersonal. It may not be suitable for you either, but if it is, it can help to control tension.

Libraries and bookshops are well stocked with books which explain, in a variety of detail, how to cope with stress. Go to your library and browse through these books. It will only cost a small amount of time, and may well be worth the trip.

An easy-to-read, commonsense approach to the subject is *Stress and Relaxation* by Jane Madders (3rd ed., Martin Dunitz, London, 1984).

Chapter Ten

THE MIRACLE DRUGS: CORTICOSTEROIDS

The discovery of corticosteroids, or steroids, as they are commonly known, was to medicine what man's first flight to the moon was to space exploration – a giant step forward for mankind. They revolutionized the treatment of disease and gave hope where little or none existed before.

The field of dermatology benefited enormously. Steroids became the drug of choice in the treatment of most non-tumorous, non-infectious skin conditions. Their use eliminated the old methods of treatment – many of which were unsightly and messy. Their use also eliminated the need to think critically about a skin problem, to evaluate and diagnose it properly. There was no need, since steroids cleared most of them up anyway. 'Give them some cortisone and it will go away,' became a common attitude. If it did not go away, then a doctor began to worry about it.

Steroids started to be used indiscriminately, and are still being used indiscriminately. This was abetted by well-meaning patients who, wishing to share their good fortune, often passed left-over medications to their friends. Use became abuse. Then came the reckoning. Side-effects began to appear, and the miracle drugs, although still pretty miraculous, lived up to the old adage that 'No one gets something for nothing'.

The steroids are still over-prescribed and overused. Who wants to wait two weeks for a rash to clear partially with a salicylic acid cream when a steroid preparation will clear it completely in less than a week? If the doctor hesitates to prescribe, the patient will probably demand it.

Since they are so prevalent in dermatological treatment, you undoubtedly have applied them to your skin, or are applying them now. In dermatitis they are a steady and frequent companion. Therefore you should know what they are, how they react on your skin and inside your body, what side-effects to look for and how to prevent them.

In 1950 a substance (Compound E, later to be known as cortisone; see Fig. 11) showed marked anti-inflammatory effects when given internally, but had no effect on the skin. It was in the chemical group called 'steroid', because of its basic three-dimensional stearic configuration. ('Stearic' refers to a fundamental crystalline form in which chemical radicals tend to create a primarily hexagonal three-dimensional structure.) Then a hydrogen atom was combined with the oxygen radical. In other words, hydroxylation of oxygen was accomplished at the C11 position of Compound E. Thus, Compound F, or hydrocortisone was formed (see Fig. 11B). It proved to be highly effective chemically and had an effect on the skin.

Scientists realized that hydrocortisone was the same as cortisol, the naturally-occurring internal hormone which is secreted by our adrenal gland and is essential for life. When hydrocortisone itself was given internally, it had several effects, many not desirable therapeutically. It suppressed the normal internal secretion of cortisol and other steroid adrenal hormones. After a short period of hydrocortisone administration, this suppression was reversible. Long periods of administration, however, would produce a prolonged suppression of natural hormone once the drug was stopped. This meant the body could not react normally when subjected to

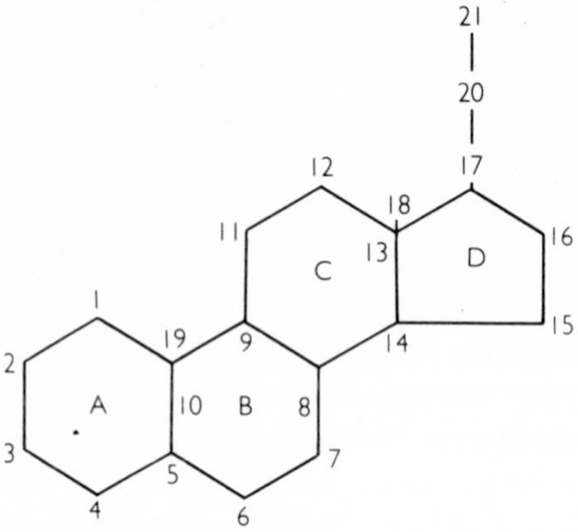

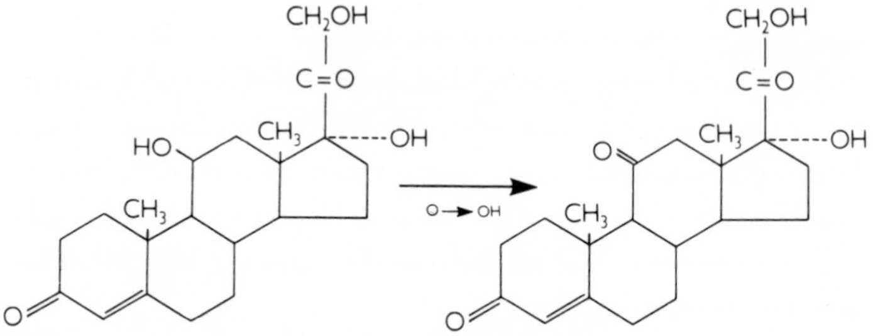

Cortisone

Hydrocortisone
(also known as Compound F
or cortisol)

Fig. 11 Basic Steroid Configurations
A Steroid skeleton.
B Comparison of cortisone and hydrocortisone.
The simple biochemical addition of hydrogen to oxygen to form the OH or hydroxyl radical transforms cortisone to hydrocortisone.

physical stress such as general infection or surgery. The result could be physiological shock.

There was also increased sodium retention which could produce oedema with accompanying potassium depletion.

The hydrocortisone, furthermore, had a major effect on glucose, protein and fat metabolism, an effect that was of no use therapeutically. In fact, it could be deleterious. Diabetes could occur with long use of hydrocortisone. Fat deposits would appear between the shoulder blades to give a 'buffalo hump' appearance. The face would round out and become moon-shaped. Wasting of muscle also developed, as well as thinning of collagen, the connective tissue substance in the dermal layer of the skin.

Two effects had beneficial therapeutic value, but could also be damaging. One was the anti-inflammatory effect due to suppression of the natural immune mechanism. This would prove extremely beneficial in many diseases, but it also masked and encouraged infection.

The second effect was inhibition of DNA synthesis within cells. This effect has proved valuable in inhibiting rapidly growing cells, such as in the plaques of psoriasis, and in raised scar tissue and in the treatment of certain leukemias and lymphomas. But in prolonged treatment, there can be an effect on normal tissue.

Armed with their knowledge, pharmaceutical chemists began an active search for a steroid that had decreased or minimal side-effects. Prednisone and prednisolone were the result. When indicated, both are commonly used in the systemic treatment of skin diseases.

TOPICAL STEROIDS

Chemical investigations were also done to find more potent topical steroids than hydrocortisone which was not as active as desired for thickened and advanced skin rashes. The addition of a fluoride radical (fluorination) to hydrocortisone at the C9 position produced several synthetic steroids (the fluorinated steroids) with enhanced potency. More manipulation of the basic steroid configuration has produced more and more potent steroids. Some have been developed with enhanced surface fat attraction which improves their penetration through the skin.

For effectiveness, topical preparations need to be available for absorption at the surface, must penetrate the skin to reach the target cells, and at the target must interact with the proper cell components in order to produce the desired effect. The newer synthetics have this ability.

They may exhibit the phenomenon of temporary insensitivity after a few days of daily use. After a few more days, however, the skin will recover and be receptive to the steroid again.

In 1961, dermatologists discovered that steroid penetration increased when the cream or ointment was used under plastic occlusion. This is simply a square of clear plastic wrap (cling film) strapped over a thick or resistant plaque to which a steroid cream has been applied. The area is then occluded for twelve to twenty-four hours.

Steroid injections directly into a thick resistant lesion also began to be used. Another means of improving steroid effectiveness was to put additives into the steroid base (vehicle) which would aid penetration. A vehicle or base is the cream or ointment into which the steroid is mixed. Sometimes the base itself aids absorption and penetration. In this regard, ointment is better than cream. The additive, propylene glycol, included with the ointment, provides further effectiveness. So does salicylic acid. Its keratolytic effect (breaking down and dissolution of scales) increases penetration. It is added to steroid preparations, but not often because of its potential as a skin irritant.

Urea was found to have hydrating (improving moisture) and keratolytic properties. Ten per cent urea is now regularly used for a steroid base. Studies have shown that the penetration of one per cent hydrocortisone in urea is twice as effective as one per cent hydrocortisone in a cream base.

Combination creams. Since infection often travels hand in hand with dermatitis, antibiotics were introduced into the steroid preparations.

Neomycin was the first of these. It has been shown to be helpful in decreasing surface bacteria, when they exist with and without overt infection. This anti-bacterial activity, in combination with a mild hydrocortisone, hastens the clearing of the dermatitis. A combination hydrocortisone/neomycin preparation works better than hydrocortisone or neomycin alone. But neomycin, if used continuously for over two weeks or sometimes for less, especially in denuded, irritated areas, can be a strong sensitizer.

Therefore, the search was on for other anti-bacterials. Hydroxyquinoline was combined with mild cortisone creams. But the use of these is falling out of favour: the quinolines stain and are themselves moderate sensitizers.

Safer topical antibiotic/corticosteroid preparations are those with tetracycline (Terra-Cortril) or erythromycin. Whether their activity is as good as neomycin's is open to challenge.

Many doctors prefer to use systemic antibiotics when indicated and avoid the topicals altogether.

Corticosteroids are also combined with anti-fungals in the treatment of yeast and other fungal infections. Yeast infections often have an acute red, moist component while other non-yeast surface fungal infections do not. Thus, anti-inflammatory effects of a mild corticosteroid are beneficial.

Nystatin is the most common anti-fungal used to treat yeast infections. Newer anti-fungals that are active against all superficial fungus infections have been developed, and can be found in combination with a mild steroid. Clotrimazole and miconazole are two of these newer multi-purpose anti-fungals.

Combination topicals, consisting of an anti-inflammatory, anti-bacterial and anti-fungal ingredient, are usually available as hydrocortisone/neomycin/nystatin preparations. Other antibiotics – polymyxin B, gramicidin – may be added in with the neomycin.

Dermatologists frown on the triple combination steroid/anti-infective therapy, seeing it as a form of 'shotgun' treatment, encouraging doctors to prescribe *carte blanche* preparations without searching for a specific cause first.

In the ano-genital area, triple creams are valuable, since both yeast and bacteria often complicate the dermatitis. Tetracycline has been substituted for neomycin, and a moderately potent corticosteroid has replaced hydrocortisone to produce trimovate, an effective cream for the ano-genital region.

The corticosteroid/anti-fungal combinations should be used primarily in acute infections where the anti-inflammatory effect is desirable to permit quicker and more efficient anti-fungal action.

Hydrocortisone is more desirable for use in combination preparations than a steroid of greater potency. There is a danger with the latter that it might 'overpower' the anti-infective action of the associated medication. In which case, the infection would not be controlled as well, and could conceivably spread.

Here are some corticosteroid/anti-infective preparations that may be prescribed for you. All, with the exception of two (trimovate and tri-adcortyl cream) have mild Group IV potency, as classified by the *British National Formulary*.

LIST 5: CORTICOSTEROID/ANTI-INFECTIVE TOPICALS

ANTI-BACTERIAL

Hydrocortisone and neomycin – 0.5 per cent of each as cream
May sensitize.

Hydroderm ointment – 1 per cent hydrocortisone (HC) and 0.5 per cent neomycin, plus bacitracin 1000 IU

Neo-cortef ointment as either 1 per cent or 2.5 per cent HC with 0.5 per cent neomycin

Neo-cortef lotion – 1 per cent HC with 0.5 per cent neomycin

Terra-cortril

ointment – 1 per cent HC and 3 per cent oxytetracycline

spray – 0.17 per cent HC and 0.5 per cent oxytetracycline

Resistant bacterial strains may develop after a period of use.

Framycort ointment – 0.5 per cent HC and 0.5 per cent framycetin

The latter ingredient has similar activity to neomycin, but no advantage. It may sensitize and cross-react with neomycin.

Genticin HC – 1 per cent HC and 0.3 per cent gentamicin

Effective, but latter ingredient sensitizes and resistant bacterial strains may develop. Use restricted.

The Quinolines

Primarily anti-bacterial with some anti-fungal effect. Stain clothing. May sensitize. Used, but not preferred.

Barquinol HC cream – 0.5 per cent HC and 3 per cent clioquinol

Vioform HC – 1 per cent HC and 3 per cent clioquinol cream and ointment

ANTI-FUNGAL

Canestan HC cream – 1 per cent HC and clotrimazole 1 per cent
For all superficial fungi.
Daktacort cream – 1 per cent HC and miconazole nitrate 2 per cent
For all superficial fungi.
Anti-yeast
Nybadex ointment – 1 per cent HC and nystatin
Nystaform HC – 0.5 per cent HC and nystatin with chlorhexidine 1 per cent cream or ointment
Chlorhexidine is an antiseptic.
Nybadex ointment – 1 per cent HC, nystatin, dimethicone 20 per cent (barrier) and benzalkonium chloride (antiseptic). Dimethicone may sensitize.
Timodine cream – 0.5 per cent HC, nystatin 100,000 IU, benzalkonium chloride 0.2 per cent

TRIPLE EFFECT

Trimovate cream – clobetasone 17 butyrate, 0.05 per cent, oxytetracycline 3 per cent (latter may cause bacterial resistance), and nystatin 100,000 IU
Clobetasone has a Class III (moderate) steroid potency.
Tri-adcortyl cream – triamcinolone acetonide (steroid with Class III activity) neomycin, gramicidin (anti-bacterial – whether it enhances activity of neomycin is not clear)
Steroxin-HC cream – 1 per cent HC, 3 per cent chlorquinaldol (a quinoline – both anti-bacterial and anti-fungal)
Stains and is moderate sensitizer.
Gregoderm ointment – 1 per cent HC, neomycin 0.4 per cent, nystatin, polymyxin B
(latter is an anti-bacterial – added because of effect against

gram negative bacteria, therefore increases potential range of anti-bacterial activity)

Terra-cortril nystatin cream – 1 per cent HC, nystatin, oxytetracycline (resistant bacterial strains may develop).

POTENCY

Topical steroid preparations are divided into four categories according to potency. The classification is basically designed to help the doctor who cannot keep up with the various corticosteroids flooding the market. In the *Formulary*, each steroid has an assigned potency grade. Thus, the doctor can pick one that is most suitable for your dermatitis.

Since side-effects do occur with these creams and ointments, it is helpful for you to know their strength too. This knowledge will make you a more intelligent user, less apt to over-medicate and more alert to possible side-effects.

According to the *British National Formulary*, the following corticosteroids with their appropriate classification are currently available for use. This list should be a handy reference for you.

LIST 6
CLASS IV – MILD POTENCY

The typical example is hydrocortisone. It is a preferred choice in mild dermatitis and in maintenance therapy after a dermatitis has been brought under control by a stronger steroid.

Hydrocortisone (HC) cream – available in strengths from 1 per cent to 0.125 per cent

Cobadex cream – 0.5 per cent or 1 per cent HC with dimethicone

Dioderm cream – 1 per cent HC

Dome-cort cream – 0.125 per cent HC

Efcortelan cream – 1 per cent or 0.5 per cent or 2.5 per cent HC

Hydrocortistab
    HC cream and ointment – 1 per cent HC

Hydrocortisyl cream and ointment – 1 per cent HC

Hydrocortisone ointment – 0.5 per cent or 1 per cent HC
    Efcortelan ointment is the same preparation.

Efcortelan ointment – 0.5 per cent, 1 per cent, 2.5 per cent HC

Hydrocortisone lotion – 1 per cent HC

Cortacream impregnated bandage – 1 per cent HC (needs strapping)

Compounds:
    Eczederm cream with 0.5 per cent HC, calamine and starch

    Epifoam – 1 per cent HC and 1 per cent pramoxine HCl in a muco-adherent base. For genital dermatitis and trauma.

    Eurax – Hydrocortisone cream – 0.25 per cent HC and 10 per cent crotamiton. (The latter is used for scabies and pruritus.)

CLASS III – MODERATELY POTENT

Fluorinated synthetic medications. Use in moderately severe or severe dermatitis, unresponsive to Class IV compounds.

Alphaderm cream – 1 per cent HC and 10 per cent urea in a powder in cream base

Calmurid HC cream – 1 per cent HC, 10 per cent urea in cream base

Ultradil plain cream and ointment – 0.1 per cent fluocortolone

Ultralanum plain cream and ointment – 0.25 per cent fluocortolone

Eumovate cream – 0.05 per cent clobetasone butyrate

Haelan cream and ointment – 0.0125 per cent flurandrenolone

CLASS II – POTENT

For severe dermatitis unresponsive to less potent steroid preparations or for chronic resistant dermatitis.

Propaderm cream and ointment – 0.025 per cent beclomethasone dipropionate

Betnovate cream and ointment – 0.1 per cent betamethasone valerate

Metosyn cream, ointment, lotion – 0.05 per cent fluocinonide cream

Haelan X cream and ointment – 0.05 per cent flurandrenolone

Adcortyl cream, ointment and spray – 0.1 per cent triamcinolone acetonide

Ledercort cream and ointment – 0.1 per cent triamcinolone acetonide

Locoid cream, ointment, scalp lotion, also as a lip cream in a fatty cream base – 0.1 per cent hydrocortisone butyrate

CLASS I – VERY POTENT

Severe dermatitis, thick chronic resistant dermatitic patches and plaques.

Halciderm cream – 0.1 per cent halcinonide

Propaderm Forte cream – 0.5 per cent beclomethasone dipropionate

Dermovate cream – 0.05 per cent clobetasol
Active in psoriasis without occlusion.

Side-effects of Topical Corticosteroids

On the whole, side-effects from topical steroids do not create a major problem. The use of these medications is well worth the risk when one considers the tremendous therapeutic benefit.

The synthetic fluorinated steroids are the most likely to cause trouble. The risk increases with the more potent substances. Plastic occlusion which enhances the penetration of steroids will also increase the risk of side-effects.

Most difficulties arise through gross abuse, either from negligence or ignorance. If you are doubtful about how to apply something, where and how to apply it, do not hesitate to ask your doctor. Left-over steroid medications should remain in your medicine cabinet and not be given to family, friends and assorted acquaintances. It is very likely that their skin problem is not the same as yours and may be made worse by the steroids.

As in most medical problems, certain people will have a greater tendency for side-effects than others. Women with fine, reddish skin can be extra-sensitive to steroid effect from preparations applied to the face. And children develop internal changes from topical applications much more so than adults. In children, the body surface area in proportion to body volume is much greater than in adults, and the potential for absorption through the skin is therefore greater.

The systemic effect of topically applied steroids can be seen in children. If steroid preparations are applied to a large body area for ten to fourteen days or longer, or if a significant proportion of the child's skin is occluded, enough steroid is absorbed to suppress the secretion of naturally occurring cortisol. However, this is not a prolonged or permanent drop. The level of cortisol will return to normal in a few days if the steroid applications cease after two weeks.

Patients, children as well as adults, who need large body areas treated for continuing periods, should have their blood cortisol levels checked about every two weeks. If tests show that there is an abnormality, then treatment should be stopped until normal levels are re-established.

The difficulty arises with chronic treatment that causes chronic suppression of the cortisol level. Then it may take a long time for the adrenal gland (and the pituitary gland which controls the adrenal) to recover. In the meantime, if the patient is put under major physical stress, such as an accident, he may go into shock. Supplemental oral steroids may be needed until the adrenal gland recovers.

In children, the systemic effect of steroids during prolonged application over a large surface may also suppress growth hormone and therefore a child's growth. This is reversible once the topical medicine is stopped.

Fortunately, internal problems from the use of topical steroids are infrequent. Nevertheless, if you need to treat large body areas on a continuing basis, you should be aware of potential hazards.

Side-effects occurring in the skin
Striae. These are the same as the stretch marks of pregnancy. Unlike stretch marks, they do not develop only on the abdomen, or just in women, and are not due to stretching. In this case, they result from the steroid's effect on the collagen in the thick elastic layer (dermis) of the skin. Over a period of time, the steroid penetrates through the epidermis in sufficient concentration to cause thinning and dissolution of the underlying collagen fibres. This undermines the support structure, permitting adjacent collagen and elastic fibres to pull the dermis apart at this weak point.

169

The result is purplish lines or striae on the skin. They are more apt to develop under plastic occlusion, especially of an extremity. Adolescents who are prone to stretch marks during their growth spurts, seem to be at higher risk of developing striae from steroids. I have seen them appear on the forearm and bend of the elbow during treatment.

Striae do not go away. The purplish colour fades with time and leaves a band of fine, crinkly skin behind.

Atrophy. The skin may become thin and shiny, and underlying small blood vessels will show in that area. Again, this occurs after prolonged use of the topicals.

After four weeks, potent preparations, under occlusion, will produce recognizable atrophy. The atrophy is secondary to a dissolution of collagen and of complex biochemicals (the ground substance) that exist between collagen fibres. There is also a thinning of the epidermis.

The skin resembles aged skin. If the steroid treatment stops, the changes will reverse, but take a long time to do so. If the atrophy has been present for a long time, the skin may never return to normal.

This atrophic skin, like ageing skin, is more prone to injury. Tiny blood vessels and capillaries in these spots are more fragile than usual. Therefore, bleeding into the skin and easy bruising occurs readily in steroid-induced atrophy.

With prolonged use of topical steroids on the face, similar changes may occur. Young women with delicate skin are most susceptible to these alterations. Often there is an obsessive quality in their pursuit of a face free from blemishes, and treatment will continue far beyond the limit.

Usually, the steroids have been prescribed for seborrhoeic dermatitis of the cheeks and around the nose, or for a mild case of adult acne. Once the problem clears, the patient continues the cream, thinking this will keep the rash from returning. Instead the skin starts to thin. Tiny blood vessels become visible, and the patient treats more vigorously, believing she sees a recurrence of her eruption. Instead, she is contributing to the development of atrophy. When she stops the applications, the original problem may rebound suddenly, requiring the use of further steroid cream to control it, but with attendant consequences. So a vicious circle begins.

If you are such a patient, it is important for the doctor to wean you off the steroids and substitute other treatment. It is best to avoid the use of potent steroids on the face of a young woman, unless the initial dermatitis is severe and unresponsive to weaker preparations.

Perioral dermatitis, or rash around the mouth, may be associated with the preceding problem. The majority of cases occur in young women who have been given strong steroids for minor facial rashes. It may also occur with applications of greasy cosmetics or creams to an already oily complexion.

In any case the eruption consists of tiny, red pustules (pimples) around the mouth, involving the chin and upper lip and nose creases. Naturally, contributory steroids or cosmetics have to be stopped.

The condition is often indolent and takes a while to clear. Treatment with a mild acne drying lotion and oral antibiotics (erythromycin or tetracycline) is usually effective.

Acne eruptions. An oily, rosy acneiform break-out is a rare complication to facial applications of hydrocortisone (Class IV) and of hydrocortisone butyrate (Class II). More commonly, regular acne pimples may arise on treated sites. Ointments and preparations under occlusion are most likely to cause this acne.

Increased hair growth may occur after repeated applications to one spot. So can mild loss of skin pigment. The latter is more common in people with dark skin.

Infections. Topical steroids should not be applied to untreated infections. They will make them worse.

Sometimes a dry, scaly patch of ringworm is inaccurately diagnosed as eczema and a corticosteroid cream will be

171

prescribed. Or you may misdiagnose it yourself and start applying a left-over steroid cream which had been effective in treatment for an old eczema.

Liberated from the body's defences by the anti-inflammatory effects of the steroid, the fungus infection will rapidly spread along the body's surface. The steroid cream may also change the appearance of the infection, making it harder to diagnose clinically.

Several times I have seen patients with extensive ringworm infections that have created unusual patterns up and down the arms, chest and back after inappropriate application of steroids. What could have initially been treated with simple topical anti-fungals now required internal medicine.

Infections are especially encouraged by the use of plastic occlusions. Pustules, caused by bacteria (staphylococci) and by yeasts, are not infrequent. Milia, or tiny sterile pustules occurring from blockage of sweat ducts under plastic occlusion, are relatively common.

Rebound phenomenon. When the suppressing effect of potent topical steroids is suddenly stopped, rashes may flare up again. The patient then has to resume the steroids and be weaned away from them gradually, either with less potent substitutes or with every other day, then every third day, and so on, steroid applications.

This is the most common side-effect, usually corrected by the gradual reduction of medication, and therefore not particularly deleterious. But there have been reports by some British doctors of an exacerbation of psoriasis, and even development of pustular psoriasis after sudden withdrawal of potent topical fluorinated steroids.

Treatment around the eye with strong steroids or with intralesional injections has to be done judiciously. Complications are rare, but are serious when they do happen. *Glaucoma* has been reported after prolonged use of the potent synthetics. If you have a pre-existing glaucoma, the use of steroids around the eye should be applied with caution, if at all.

Intralesional steroid injections into chronic skin conditions near the eye have on rare occasions resulted in sudden *blindness*. The injected fluid, inadvertently, entered the circulation and travelled to the central retinal artery where it caused a blockage.

Also, injections into the scalp, near or above the forehead, may enter lymphatics coursing downwards across the forehead and cause atrophy of skin along the branch of the lymphatic vessel.

Allergic contact dermatitis may be produced by the topical steroid itself, although this is rare, or by the preservative in the base, or by the base itself. In the latter two instances, the steroid may mask some of the allergic reaction.

However, if corticosteroids are used sensibly and appropriately in skin therapy, side-effects can be greatly minimized or avoided. You will then be able comfortably to get the most benefit from this important group of drugs.

Chapter Eleven

CONCLUSIONS

'Your patients never die and they never get better' – that is a comment frequently made to dermatologists by doctors in other specialities. The statement is delivered in a tone of humorous indictment. The implication is that if a doctor's patients 'never die' then he or she is not treating seriously ill patients and, therefore, cannot be a serious doctor. And if they 'never get better', then he or she cannot be any good either – otherwise everyone would be cured.

The phrase is certainly full of irony. Would any humane doctor want dead patients haunting his or her memories? Certainly not.

Actually, dermatologists are a fortunate breed. I think recognition of this by other doctors prompts a certain resentment and envy, which encourages other specialists to react to skin doctors as they do. It is rewarding and relaxing for a doctor not to have life and death worries, and to know that the patient's risk of dropping dead from his dermatitis is decidedly less than his chance of getting hit by a car while crossing King's Road in Chelsea.

The 'never get better' part of the phrase is the one that bothers me. It implies an inability to heal – and what doctor worth his or her salt does not want to heal a patient? It is the main joy in practising medicine. Yet in dermatology, diseases are chronic. The skin may look clear, but that does not mean it is cured and that the doctor can joyfully bid goodbye to the patient. In fact, the doctor and patient may see a lot of each other through the coming years.

As the skin eruption goes through periods of remission and relapses, the patient begins to look at the doctor with reproach, or the doctor begins to think the patient is looking at him or her with reproach. 'Why can't you cure me, doctor?' seems to be written large in his eyes. The guilt of the doctor may be conveyed to the patient and the patient's frustration may be conveyed to the doctor. Pressure rises for stronger medications and new, unproven methods – often to the disadvantage of the patient.

The treatment of a chronic illness demands a partnership between the patient and doctor. The doctor needs to accept his or her limitations, and acknowledge that although there may be no cure, there is much that can be done to improve the patient's skin and quality of life. This information should not be buried deep within the doctor's bosom, but should be shared with the patient, who can then begin to get involved with his or her own care.

We should not become dismayed by chronic, recurrent skin conditions and the inability to make them vanish for ever with a magical medicine. There are many other medical problems that have no 'cure' as such. How many cases of headaches, stomach ulcers and nervous bowel disorders are actually cured? Not one of them. The potential for these stress-induced disorders exists throughout the patient's life.

And so in dermatology. To cure skin diseases we have to get at the source, but in our present state of knowledge we really do not know the specific mechanism responsible for the majority of these conditions.

But if we cannot 'cure', in the sense that something will clear and never return, we can certainly control and prevent dermatitis.

The most successful doctor is not only sympathetic and understanding, but also relaxed, thoughtful and open with his or her patients. He or she should be able to admit general medical ignorance about a problem, yet remain hopeful and positive about its outcome. Hope is a very important aspect, not only of healing, but of surviving in life. We have all heard the words, 'born loser', in reference to someone who is never able to achieve his goals or to accomplish something for himself. I do not like the phrase very much. As a matter of fact, I do not like it at all. It comes down as an indictment, a dogmatic assumption, and the book is closed on someone. No one is 'born' to lose. Our surroundings, the attitudes of our family, and of other people close to us early in life, determine how we react and how we perceive ourselves. If we are always told we are no good, inadequate and will never do anything, we begin to believe it, whether we walk around sullen and depressed, or belligerently begin to react against these feelings.

If you, the patient, have attitudes of hopelessness and dejection, or thoughts such as 'this will never get better', or 'I'll never be able to do that', you will have a difficult time improving your state of health. Cast off such attitudes. Seek out people who are positive, who give you positive reinforcement. Continuing negative attitudes can be self-fulfilling, but so can positive ones.

It is important to keep that in mind when thinking about your skin problems. Be hopeful, stay positive – actively work at these attitudes. There is little reason why you should not improve and stay well if you set your mind to it.

From time to time one reads amazing stories of people in whom cancer has gone into 'spontaneous' remission. These are usually people who adopt forceful, positive attitudes towards their illness, towards life and, therefore, manage to prevail.

We know about yoga practitioners who with dedication,

time and practice, are able to control their breathing, heart rate, blood pressure, even their tendency to bleed. All of these mechanisms are controlled by our autonomic nervous system, the same system that controls responses in the skin. It stands to reason that if one can control internal functions through the nervous system, one should also be able to improve skin functions. For it is likely that our body defences, such as our immune system, can be improved by our mental state which influences the neural-hormonal response that affects our immunology.

Recently I read in *The Times* about two young men who remarkably brought AIDS under control. Both had been very ill and were expected to die. Each decided he would fight back and not succumb to the disease. One of them stopped his chemotherapy, which was making him sick, and left the hospital. Both began to change their mental attitudes. They refused to give in to despair and hopelessness. They thought positively about cure. At the same time they began a highly nutritious diet and a regimen of rest and exercise.

One of the men mentally concentrated on his AIDS skin tumour, willing its regression, imagining it diminishing to nothing. He did this day after day, determined to succeed, while maintaining his exercises and diet. At the end of six months, the tumour was gone and there was no evidence of active AIDS in his bloodstream. The change did not come easily to this man. It took commitment, determination and positive conviction – all important elements in successfully executing any project.

This is a dramatic example of what can be done to improve health if you 'set your mind to it'. If this man could control a deadly illness, then you should be able to control a common one that is not life-threatening.

A valuable contribution to good health, mental and physical, is humour. 'A merry heart works like a doctor', and 'Laughter is the music of life' are literate versions of 'Laughter is the best medicine'. Do not go through life gloomy, morose or angry about how life is treating you. Instead, you should ask, 'How am I treating life?' Maintain a sense of humour about yourself, your skin problem and about life around you. There is humour even in the most dreary and seemingly insufferable daily circumstances. The writer Chekhov, a victim of consumption which in his time was incurable, was a master at illuminating that aspect of human interaction.

By all means, if you are in an insufferable work or personal situation, take positive steps to change it. But while you are going about these changes, try not to dwell on your troubles. Try this. At this moment – think of a good joke or funny situation. It will make you smile and you will feel better.

Norman Cousins, who was editor of the *Saturday Review* for many years, wrote a book, *Anatomy of an Illness,* about how humour helped him overcome a crippling arthritic disease of his spine. Several doctors told him there was no cure, and that he had to resign himself to lifelong pain, medication and eventual deformity of the spine.

Cousins rejected his doctors' prognosis and decided to cure himself. With the co-operation of an understanding doctor, he submerged himself in humour and took large doses of Vitamin C. He had read that it might have merit in his disease. During this period of several weeks, he watched film comedies (Groucho Marx, Charlie Chaplin), and read many humorous books – Mark Twain, Stephen Leacock, etc. At the end of his medical retreat he emerged healthy and has stayed well.

Cousins did not start this regimen blindly. He had an intelligent knowledge of his disease, of the use of Vitamin C in its treatment, and of the effects of laughter on one's health.

Knowledge is the first step towards prevention. Doctors and nurses can help to educate you, and even guide you to the point of beginning prevention, but the actual prevention of your illness is by and large up to you. Preventive medicine depends on how strong your desire is to implement the information which has been imparted to you.

I hope this book will provide the first important step, and that you will take the second.

INDEX

INDEX